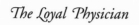

The Loyal Physician

The Loyal Physician

ROYCEAN ETHICS AND THE
PRACTICE OF MEDICINE

Griffin Trotter

VANDERBILT UNIVERSITY PRESS
Nashville & London

First edition 1997
97 98 99 00 01   5 4 3 2 1

This publication is made from recycled paper and meets
the minimum requirements of American National Standard for Information Sciences—
Permanence of Paper for Printed Library Materials ∞

Library of Congress Cataloging-in-Publication Data

Trotter, Griffin, 1957-
    The loyal physician : Roycean ethics and the practice of medicine
/ Griffin Trotter. -- 1st ed.
      p.   cm. -- (The Vanderbilt library of American philosophy)
    Includes bibliographical references and index.
    ISBN 0-8265-1291-7
    1. Physicians--Professional ethics. 2. Loyalty. 3. Royce,
Josiah, 1855-1916. 4. Physicians--Conduct of life. 5. Medical
ethics.   I. Title. II. Series.
    R725.5.T76 1997
    174'.2--dc21   97-4638
                                                                                            CIP

Manufactured in the United States of America

To my mother and father:
whenever I write of loyalty, I refer to them

Contents

Acknowledgments

Among my numerous mentors who deserve thanks for their assistance with this project, John Lachs stands out. My work has been repeatedly nurtured and transfused—as well as rescued from folly—by his boundless reservoir of wisdom, energy, and dedication. His capacity for dosing laughter and joy in the context of penetrating philosophical expositions is legendary at Vanderbilt University, as witnessed by the waiting lists for his courses in ethics and the ubiquitous clamor for his services as a public speaker. In six years as his student, I have called on him countless times—for guidance, for expert commentary, and for friendly support. He has never failed me.

It would be impossible to thank adequately the many other educators and friends whose contributions stand behind this effort (but who should not be blamed for its shortcomings). Special thanks go to John Stuhr, Kenneth Iserson, Jeffrey Tlumak, Michael Hodges, Richard Zaner, George Ball, and Frank Oppenheim for their philosophical guidance. The late Tony Andrews, of Emanuel Hospital in Portland, Oregon, and Vallee Willman, of St. Louis University, deserve accolades as clinical instructors. So do several friends and colleagues, especially Fr. Jim Tobin, Ragnar Storaasli, Kirk Anderson, Dan Wascher, Dale Siner, Sighla Kujawa, Kathy Gullick, Jerry Evans, Michelle Williams, and Dan Kingsberry.

My wife Candyce, and our sons—Orion, Shane, and little Griffin—have endured more trials than anyone on behalf of this book. I cannot thank them enough. Many other family members also deserve recognition, but the list is too long for inclusion here. Amy Guy, my sister, must be the exception. She is in many ways the finest example I know of the loyal personality.

And, finally, I want to thank my parents and my patients. Under the watchful eye of my mother and father, I lived a childhood full of love, security, warmth, challenge, and adventure. Whatever good I make of my life, I owe to these wonderful early years. In the last fourteen years, it is perhaps my patients who are most responsible for helping me to preserve that sense of wonder that characterizes youth, and to continue to grow. Thank you, Mr. Tinajero, Mrs. Louthen, Mr. Henson, and countless others. Without you, this book would have been groundless and pointless.

List of Abbreviations for Cited Works

All works are by Royce, unless otherwise noted.
For full bibliographic information, see Bibliography.

AV	*After Virtue,* by Alisdair MacIntyre
CG	*The Conception of God*
ECE	1915–1916 Extension Course in Ethics *
HGC	*The Hope of the Great Community*
HS	Herbert Spencer
LHE	Lectures in the History of Ethics *
LJR	*The Letters of Josiah Royce*
OP	*Outlines of Psychology*
PC	*The Problem of Christianity*
PL	*The Philosophy of Loyalty*
RAP	*The Religious Aspect of Philosophy*
RLE	*Royce's Logical Essays*
RPL	Royce's Pittsburgh Lectures *
RQP	*Race Questions and Other American Problems*
RUL	*Royce's Urbana Lectures,* Lecture 2
SGE	*Studies in Good and Evil*
SRI	*The Sources of Religious Insight*
WAR	*War and Insurance*
WI	*The World and the Individual*
WJE	*William James and other Essays on the Philosophy of Life*
WJWR	*Whose Justice, Which Rationality,* by Alisdair MacIntyre

* Unpublished works of Royce found in Harvard University Archives, Royce Papers (see Bibliography)

❖

Introduction

■ It is easy enough to say that man is immortal simply because he will endure: that when the last ding-dong of doom has clanged and faded from the last worthless rock hanging tideless in the last red and dying evening, that even then there will still be one more sound: that of his puny inexhaustible voice, still talking. I refuse to accept this. I believe that man will not merely endure: he will prevail. He is immortal, not because he alone among creatures has an inexhaustible voice, but because he has a soul, a spirit capable of compassion and sacrifice and endurance. The poet's, the writer's, duty is to write about these things. It is his privilege to help man endure by lifting his heart, by reminding him of the courage and honor and hope and pride and compassion and pity and sacrifice which have been the glory of his past. The poet's voice need not merely be the record of man, it can be one of the props, the pillars to help him endure and prevail.

—William Faulkner

A midst the skepticism and misanthropy of the late twentieth century, Faulkner's words seem out-of-step, as though the utterer sought to reinstitute a wrongheaded order of rackety spiritual anthems and beckoning Holy Grails. Somehow, he seems to have missed the lesson of two world wars—and likely would have missed the later lessons of Viet Nam—that passionate belief in the dignity of humankind is, in reality, a mask for cultural imperialism. In contemporary thought, there is a new axiom: "Philanthropy and moral idealism always have a dark side." With it comes a new maxim: "The grand motives of so-called humanitarians are properly objects only of derision, or disinterest, or deconstruction." The narratives of postmodernism have no place of honor for illustrious missions and sweeping moral visions, except in the contracted sense in which the life and work of the cynic is, indeed, glorified. Curiously, for one so attuned to humanity's inhumanity, Faulkner stands outside this orthodoxy—clueless, as it were.

Josiah Royce was similarly beguiled. Royce calls us, as passionately as Faulkner, to take up the mantle of human honor and decency. For Royce, the elevation of humanity is a vocation belonging to everyone—to poets, novelists, statesmen, and philosophers, but also to soldiers, laborers, homemakers, and professionals. All are responsible, in Royce's view, for the augmentation of the human spirit. All are called to toil upon the scaffolds of Royce's towering ideal—the "Great Community" of all humanity. Though he was as attuned to evil as any philosopher of his day, Royce—like Faulkner—misses the seemingly necessary link between moral idealism and spiritual degradation.

One of the aims of this work is to reclaim the spirit of these latter day Quixotes and see how it fares in the world of modern medicine. We will suppose, for awhile, that a moral life is something grand. And we will look to Royce for guidance about how to live it. We will be serious about moral traditions, examining our own and asking how the moral life might be restored to a place of honor.

Such an undertaking will require that we be skeptical about the current skepticism, and consider, at least momentarily, that beneath a veneer of cynicism and aloofness, the modern intellectual may have sequestered something vital. We will ask whether the voice of moral idealism may itself be one of history's recent casualties and whether it might be worth hearing.

In an era of spiritual malaise, such an undertaking will require uncommon diligence. Should we become serious about idealistic prescriptions, we are in for a monumental struggle. Royce tells us that those who undertake to live a moral life must be willing to suffer. They must safeguard a humble recognition of their own fallibility and of their measly defenses against threats of deception, moral decrepitude, and desperation. They must be vigorous and thoroughgoing, transfusing the pale corpus of daily routine with the lifeblood of their calling. These requirements are summarized by Royce in the notion of loyalty.

I believe the modern provider of health care would benefit from grappling with Royce. No physician, no nurse, no hospital administrator could read *The Philosophy of Loyalty* and not be affected. As one of their rank, I have felt Royce's challenge. The health-care community is under siege. We have been distracted by a din of voices that question our integrity, our humanity, and our role within the larger community. Royce would tell us that we have no one to blame but ourselves. We must impeach ourselves, not because of any cumulative responsibility for the evils of medicine but because we have listened too unreflectively to the lamentations of our critics. We have allowed our community to become infected by the selfishness and moral apathy of society at large. Beneath our accusers' demands for technical flawlessness and cost-effectiveness—readily enough perceived as contradictory—runs a current of spiritual bankruptcy. Engaged as we are in the debate over particulars, we are drawn in without a struggle by this subterranean influence.

Royce challenges us to take the hard path of a higher calling. We should, in his view, demand more of ourselves than could be reasonably expected. We should contribute more than people have a right to receive. We should be our own harshest critics. And we should take pains to ensure that the reconstruction of our professional lives occurs on moral high ground, informed by a consistent loyalty to humanitarian ideals, rather than in the snake pit of partisan politics informed only by the conflicting imperatives of confused moral relativism.

Of course, warnings about the precarious state of humanitarianism in medicine have been issued for decades. In the late 1950s, several studies documented how the outlooks of medical students became increasingly cynical and decreasingly benevolent during medical school (Fox 1957; Becker and Geer 1958; Christie and Merton 1958; Eron 1958). By 1974 there was enough literature on the subject for Rezler to draw it together in a review article. One of her conclusions was that detachment from broad humanitarian concerns was so prominent among clinical faculty that the initial positive effects of special programs designed to stimulate social values in students were consistently lost during the course of clinical clerkships (Rezler 1974, 1029). In 1992, Colwill observed, with ample documentation, that young physicians exhibited increasing degrees of self-centeredness, especially with regard to financial gain, and that this trend was not merely a reflection of changing social attitudes about morality but was also cultivated by the peculiarities of training in the academic medical center. Within the context of such a decline in the moral consciousness of medical professionals, it is no surprise that the humanitarian foundations of medical practice have also been eroded. From the vantage point of medical entrepreneurs, the moral tradition in medicine has largely been neglected—seen as irrelevant, overly demanding or archaic. From the vantage point of those who are concerned about medicine's inability to meet the needs of the public, the tradition has been challenged—seen as contradictory, self-serving, or, once again, archaic.

What emerges from all this conflict is a kind of institutional identity crisis. The medical profession, challenged by critics and reformers, is hard-pressed to give account of itself. Just what do we stand for? What do we revere? Where are we headed? These questions are becoming increasingly important yet increasingly difficult to answer. Our paralysis in the face of such questions and challenges is the central problem around which this book was written.

This problem is a moral problem. Like most moral problems, it has several components. First, there is a psychological problem, rooted, Royce would tell us, in the psychological need for a coherent personal identity. The lack of such an identity manifests itself in a feeling of incompleteness. Most of us seek to integrate our profession into a whole life and are therefore concerned with our professional identities. Without the support of a coherent tradition, the cultivation of a professional identity is difficult. The professional who lacks a clear sense of his or her mission and role in society is likely to feel anxious and vulnerable before a multitude of assaults from outside the profession. Further, we must deal with what Peirce calls "the irritation of doubt." Questions about the task of medicine are real ones. The absence of beliefs about the answers is itself a psychological problem.

Second, there is an epistemological problem, parented by the irritation of doubt. It is a problem about the fixation of belief. It consists in our lack of a procedure for identifying which claims about the tasks or ideals of medicine are worthy of our assent. We will not be satisfied with just any tradition, with just any structure for organizing our ideals. We want to live in accord with the truth, and, therefore, we need to learn how we learn about the truth.

Third, there is a metaphysical problem, which consists of the fact that, even given the epistemological procedure we seek, we cannot yet know where it will take us. The task of formulating and serving ideals is complicated. It is arduous, and it is an eternal challenge. Further, we are never guaranteed of our virtuosity in applying our method of fixating beliefs. Even when we walk in the spirit of truth, our conception of specifics may be erroneous.

The division of moral problems into psychological, epistemological, and metaphysical components is somewhat artificial. According to Royce and other pragmatists, we cannot have one without the others; they overlap. Nevertheless, it is worth noting that Royce gives each of these problems some individual attention. In *The Philosophy of Loyalty*, for instance, Royce begins with a psychological problem and approaches the other two only in light of the former. In *The Sources of Religious Insight* and "The Principles of Logic," Royce addresses primarily epistemological issues. In *The World and the Individual*, Royce's fundamental concern is with metaphysics.

Our approach in this essay will combine elements of Royce's approaches in *The Problem of Christianity* and *The Philosophy of Loyalty*. In PC, Royce begins with a general question which has direct psychological, epistemological, and metaphysical bearings. He asks, "In what sense, if any, can the modern man consistently be, in creed, a Christian?" (PC, 62). The central question of this essay is analogous and could be formulated as, In what sense, if any, can the modern physician consistently be, in creed, a loyalist? We will study the current state of medicine and discover an array of difficult challenges, some being of a relatively unprecedented nature. Hearkening to these challenges, we will turn to Royce's philosophy of loyalty.

Our investigation will be analogous to *The Philosophy of Loyalty* in that we will begin with the analysis of a psychological problem—specifically the aforementioned problem of professional identity. It will be portrayed as both an institutional and an individual problem. Therefore our sense of "psychological" will be rather expansive, combining strands of traditional psychology with what could be classified as sociology. Royce integrates these areas well.

To treat the psychological problem adequately , we will need to discuss several epistemological and metaphysical issues. We will avoid, however, an expansive treatment of Royce's metaphysics. Further, we will extricate Royce's moral theory from Royce's theology whenever this seems feasible, and we will refrain from attempting a complete chronological development of Royce's ethical theory. These points are important to the purpose and centeredness of this essay. Excellent historical accounts of Royce's ethics (Fuss 1965; Oppenheim 1993) and Royce's theology (Jarvis 1975; Oppenheim 1987) are already available. Our mission in this essay is different. We want to respond to some major contemporary problems in the philosophy of medicine by developing important aspects of Royce's thought and investigating how they might be helpful for the problems at hand. As such an enterprise, the essay aims to be a kind of prolonged dialogue between Royce and modern medicine, with the author acting as a kind of intermediary. The author's mission, then, is to embody, as much as possible, that peculiar form of the spirit of interpretation that potentiates a fruitful "interpretive musement" of the variety championed by Royce and Peirce (Oppenheim 1987, 264–279; Oppenheim 1993, 127–132). The concern in such an undertaking is not with the chronological development, or even with the comprehensive summation, of a moral theory. Instead, successful interpretive musement conducts a favorable interplay between various leading ideas (ideas having broad, general implications and seemingly great heuristic potential but that cannot themselves be directly confirmed as to their value or truthfulness). An example would be Royce's 1915–1916 Extension Course in Ethics, where he developed a deep and nuanced appreciation of several of the great themes in ethics by treating each of three central "leading ideas of ethics": autonomy, goodness, and duty. In that same series of lectures, Royce developed his general notion of loyalty by looking at three species of family loyalty and by viewing each within the context of these three leading ideas.

To refrain from summarizing a corpus of moral doctrine is *not* to reject the theoretical imperatives for adequately grounding one's moral ideas and for ensuring their mutual coherence. Our response to these theoretical imperatives is the reason we will not be able to refrain altogether from doing metaphysics or epistemology. On the other hand, I think it is quite possible to sketch a Roycean moral theory and to show how it is defensible, without delineating the evolution of each Roycean moral idea within a historical account of Royce's philosophical development. For many of the purposes of this essay, the subtle differences characterizing each of the successive stages of Royce's philosophical development are either irrelevant or too far afield of our objectives to warrant comment. Thus, I have no qualms about drawing from early sources such as LHE and RAP within the context of a discussion of later works, as long as our heuristic objectives are not compromised. As Royce himself has commented (PC 350), most of the changes that characterize his later works, such as PC, are changes in emphasis or "mode of approach" and do not represent significant reversals or amendments of his previous positions. Sometimes these changes will be important for our objectives. In these cases, they will be underscored. When they are not important, they will frequently be passed over without comment.

The greatest potential stumbling block for this project is, perhaps, the challenge of fairly representing Royce without attending in great depth to his theology. My purpose for taking this non-theological approach is simple—I seek to reach a diverse audience, which includes many who would not be receptive to (and some who would be repelled by) religious philosophy in general or Christian doctrine in particular. Nevertheless, Royce *was* a Christian thinker, a fact that cannot be ignored if we are to understand him. At several junctures, we will, of necessity, refer to Royce's religious thought. Often, it will be possible for readers, if they so desire, to reinterpret fruitfully these aspects of Royce's work in non-Christian terms. I think, in fact, that the Roycean theory of medical ethics developed here should be appealing to thinkers from a variety of religious backgrounds, including atheism. To this end, I am willing (provisionally) to attenuate Royce's religious message. My hope is that I do not, in this endeavor, diminish Royce to the point that I am doing him, and my readers, a disservice.

We will speak of a "grand tradition" in medicine, referring to a loosely organized conglomerate of several traditions having cumulatively held sway in modern medicine, at least until the last few decades. The term *tradition,* used with reference to the profession of medicine, will refer to the customs, principles, and arguments that characterize a relatively coherent and continuous, historically extended way of professional life. The grand tradition, we will find, traces itself to a complex moral ancestry. Because the various ancestor traditions that combine in the "grand tradition" come from relatively independent, irreconcilable sources, we stretch our definition of *tradition* when we take the grand tradition as a single entity. We are not alone, however, in this endeavor.[1] There are as many versions of the grand tradition as there are commentators who seek to formulate it. Yet, there is much that the various accounts have in common. A heuristic unification of medicine's diverse traditions is, I believe, both tenable and fruitful.

The working hypothesis of this essay is that the identity problems afflicting medicine—that is, the deficiencies in medicine's grand tradition—may be remedied with the help of Josiah Royce's philosophy of loyalty. I will attempt to show that the notion of genuine loyalty is an adequate and desirable basis for the development of a coherent medical ethics. It is a suitable basis, I will show, not merely for a "professional ethic" in the narrow sense developed by Veatch (1981, 82), where it would be accessible only to professionals, but also for a comprehensive social ethics of medicine, accessible to nonprofessionals as well. Since the "identity crisis" of medicine is a problem for society at large, and not merely for doctors or other health professionals, the solution to this problem must be suitable to the larger group as well as to the professional group.

It is quite natural to begin a treatment of Royce's philosophy with questions of personal and group identity.[2] Because the Roycean conception of an intact tradition is subservient to the notion of a healthy community, it also makes sense to begin an inquiry such as ours with the discussion of personal identity, then moving to the notion of community, then to the tradition.

Royce's notes from his Pittsburgh Lecture contain an impressive summary of his association of loyalty with personal identity:

> Tell me to what you are loyal, and why,—and you tell me at once just what constitutes the really moral aspect of your personality. All the rest is chance, or fortune, or prejudice or barren routine. Tell me, again, wherein and whereto you are loyal, and you will at once explain to me how far you have personally solved the problem about the conflict between personal rights and social duties. (RPL 1:24–25)

For Royce, selfhood arises out of a plan for life and is constituted by the enactment of a plan. Much like Aristotle, Royce sees the good life as activity directed by and toward an ideal or *telos*. Royce holds that a personal ideal—one that establishes one's identity—must have two characteristics: (1) it must provide the individual with a means of differentiating himself from others, and (2) it must impart to the individual a sense of continuity. Achieving (1) interferes with achieving (2) insofar as self-differentiation is identified with self-sufficiency. This pitfall is avoided if we recognize that self-differentiation does not occur in isolation. It happens in the context of community membership. Since the achievement of continuity is impossible apart from some sort of social structure (for example, having a name, having a role, having a language, being able to expect relatively uniform treatment in like circumstances, and so forth), the individual who perceives the task of self-differentiation to be the task of extricating himself from social influence is bound to end up in what Royce called "the solipsism of the present moment," where there is no continuity.

Such an individual is confronted with a central paradox—what we shall term "the paradox of self-realization." He is the self-appointed master of his own moral destiny, but, by himself, he is not able to establish even a hint of moral continuity. What is called for if we are to resolve the paradox, according to Royce, is an outlook that reconciles individualistic needs for self-differentiation with communitarian needs for structure and affiliation. He investigates several ideals—the hero, the self-denying self, and the rebel—by which human beings have, historically, attempted to achieve such a reconciliation. Each of these ideals is found to have peculiar strengths but also to be deficient in one way or another. In the light of these failures, Royce offers the ideal of loyalty—conceived as the willing, thoroughgoing and practical devotion to a cause—which he finds to combine the strengths of the others, without the shortcomings.

We will follow Royce through this line of reasoning. Then, when we come to the conclusion that loyalty exceeds other personality ideals, we will ask, How, and in what sense, is the ideal of loyalty morally compelling? This question will lead us into the realm of Royce's "moral insight." This moral insight, simple in nature but complicated in its ramifications, occurs when we expand our realm of consciousness so as to understand the world from the perspective of those other than ourselves

(not just in the sense of sharing feelings but in the manner of provisionally willing what they will). To understand the force of the moral insight,
we will have to be familiar with Royce's theory of interpretation.

One effect of the moral insight is the realization that the ideal of each
individual is valid prima facie and that any moral theory worth its salt will
be one that maximizes the possibilities for reconciling and harmonizing
competing ideals. This line of thinking will lead us to the conclusion that
we ought, as much as possible, to harmonize our loyalties. Royce summarizes this requirement in his notions of loyalty to loyalty, as well as loyalty to the great community (a harmonious community of all humanity).
Genuine loyalty occurs, in Royce's view, when we subordinate natural loyalties to these higher loyalties.

After developing the theory of loyalty, we will turn to medicine and
begin with a discussion of the physician-patient relation. Though this relation is classically taken as the fundamental molecule from which the edifice of professional medical ethics is constructed, we will find that the
obligations that attend it are engendered from higher obligations. Both
the physician and the patient are members of a larger community—what
I will call the greater medical community (GMC)—which includes clinicians, other frontline or adjunctive health professionals, researchers, patients, and potential patients. The GMC arises from a shared devotion to
public health. It is a community because each of its members has a part
in serving and defining its central ideal. Unlike the medical community,
conceived as a professional community, membership in the GMC is open
to the public.

We will discover how the physician-patient relation, taken by itself, is
inherently unstable. This instability, we will find, can be mediated by an
appeal to the GMC. We will traverse some of the intricate workings of the
GMC and eventually conclude that the physician, like the patient, ought
to conceive of loyalty to the physician-patient relation as a function of
one's loyalty to the GMC, placing that loyalty to the GMC under the loyalty to the great community. Further, the professional community, instead
of being a kind of trade union, as many now conceive it, should be devoted entirely to the ideals of the GMC. The "self-interest" of medical
professionals should be aligned with the general ideal of the GMC—that
is, with the health of the public—and thus should not conflict with the
interests of patients.

We will explore several important implications of this view. First, we will find that the classic tension between egoism and altruism is mitigated by the physician's personal commitment to community ideals. We will also discover a natural basis for the commitment to patient autonomy, while seeing that this commitment is not medicine's defining ideal. Third, we will discover that, though the physician's highest professional obligation is to the GMC, the best strategy for honoring this obligation is usually for the physician to strive to meet the needs of individual patients. Fourth, we will find that the "entrepreneurial model" of medical practice—where the physician is conceived as one whose primary aim is profit—is destructive to loyalty and ought to be reviled. Our attitude toward entrepreneurialism, however, will not lead us to condemn the free market, and, thus, we will be critical of government intervention in health care. Fifth, we will examine various notions of the "gatekeeper role" in medicine, finding that the use of physician gatekeepers is, on occasion, justified but only because of a discouragingly widespread lack of commitment to community ideals. In general, we will follow Pellegrino and Thomasma in a critique of this role.

Many criticisms will be brought against the current practice of medicine and the current practices of established medical associations. Because of the breadth of the subject matter, most of these criticisms will be brief and suggestive. The final chapter will present, by the help of specific metaphors, an overview of the relation of loyalty to such subvirtues as honesty and courage.

I believe our treatment of Royce is important, first of all, because of the failure of previous attempts at formulating a comprehensive theory of medical ethics. We will discuss, albeit briefly, where I think some of these competing theories go awry. In comparison to the alternatives, Royce's doctrine of loyalty has several important merits that recommend it to medicine. These include: (1) the manner in which it responds to the broad range of problems that arise in the day-to-day life of health-care providers and patients, not confining itself to "sticky situations"; (2) its attentiveness to the cultivation of character rather than mere adherence to moral rules; (3) the manner in which it mediates fragmentizing influences predominating in other theories; and (4) its openness to various interpretations. Ultimately, I think Royce's theory is the best foundation for medical ethics because it is philosophically the strongest among its competitors.

A second important contribution of Royce's addresses the broader social problem of reconciling individualism with commitment to community service. This issue is currently front and center in the national consciousness. Royce can, I believe, shed considerable light in this area. If I am right, the study of his theory will be worthwhile for this reason alone.

Third, this essay represents the first comprehensive treatment of professional medical ethics using the tools of a classical American philosopher. Though my efforts will, no doubt, fall short of what these thinkers themselves might have achieved, it is important that someone start the ball rolling. Much of distinct value within the American philosophic tradition awaits the kind of consideration I am proposing, and to neglect its relevance to professional ethics is unconscionable. Royce commented in PL that his theory provides a template for a professional ethic (PL, 21); yet eighty-eight years later not a single attempt has been made to follow up on this claim.

The neglect of Royce, I believe, is based largely on ignorance. While contemporaries such as Peirce, Dewey, and James have received at least a modicum of attention, Royce has been unfairly branded as the American reincarnation of Hegel. Anyone who finishes this essay will know that this label is unjust. Further, while Royce's metaphysics departs sharply on several issues from Hegel's, his ethics departs rather radically from how he himself has come to be interpreted by several casual readers. In this regard, Royce's fate is reminiscent of that of a kindred spirit—the Italian patriot Giuseppe Mazzini.

Mazzini wrote, in *The Duties of Man*, that "You are men before you are citizens or fathers." Like Royce, he was careful to subordinate national loyalties to a higher loyalty to all humanity. Nevertheless, Mazzini wrote passionately about the duties of citizens, and, in the words of Greer, "Ironically, many of his readers, then and later, became so attentive to the glory of the nation that they forgot his precept of a prior duty to humanity" (Greer 1982, 430–431). Likewise, Mazzini's emphasis on the primacy of individual freedom was lost in the nationalist fervor that came to be associated with his work. Thus, Mazzini's invocations have been associated with fascism and aggressive nationalism in Italian politics, quite in contrast to the spirit in which they were put forth.

Royce never enjoyed the public attention bestowed on Mazzini. But, probably because of a too-facile association of his theory with the ideas of public figures such as Theodore Roosevelt (whom he disliked, though, admittedly, with whom he had much in common), Royce has come to be discredited. A fallibilist, he is often called a dogmatist. He was always concerned to derive and illustrate the practical implications of his theories, yet is often portrayed as a proponent of barren, remote abstractions. Though he continually stressed that the key to a thriving community is the cultivation of individual differences, he is frequently written off as the enemy of freedom and individuality. As Cornel West has rightly pointed out, no American philosopher was as deeply respectful of the problem of evil as Royce (West 1993, 113–118). Yet Royce's own friend and colleague, William James, accused him of creating a "block universe," which blotted out the flesh-and-blood world of moral ambiguity and human suffering.

It is interesting that one of Royce's devoted students and friends, Richard Clark Cabot, had an important role in the metamorphosis of modern medical ethics. It may well be that Royce's greatest (or only) influence on medicine has been through Cabot. Not surprisingly, Cabot has also been misunderstood. Though he subordinated his recommendations about the application of technology to his understanding of larger issues about the welfare of the public, he has come to be associated with the doctrine that the competent application of technology is a good in itself. In the cases of both Royce and Cabot, as with Mazzini, the characteristics that caused their ideas to go out of fashion were more in the nature of accretions applied by unenlightened interpreters than they were tenets of their respective philosophies. To my knowledge, no informed thinker has ever offered an earnest attempt to refute the basic principles of Royce's philosophy of loyalty.

There are several limitations to this essay that deserve notice. First, when we speak of medicine's irreconcilable ancestor traditions, a question arises about whether the traditions are incommensurable or merely incompatible. We will assume the ancestor traditions are commensurable. To a large degree, our project may be viewed as the task of developing an adequate theory by which they may be mediated.[3]

Second, there are two important ways in which my account of professional medical ethics is biased. I speak repeatedly about physicians, and rarely about nurses, technicians, hospital administrators, and other members of the health-care team. Also, I fashion an overwhelming preponder-

ance of examples, issues, and cases from the practice of emergency medicine, generally to the neglect of other specialties. The most obvious reason for these biases is that I am a physician specializing in emergency
medicine. It is important to me that my analysis be grounded in firsthand
experience. I also believe that emergency medicine is sorely neglected in
most discussions of professional medical ethics and deserves emphasis.
The result is that I have more regrets about excluding nurses and technicians from my account than I do about slighting other specialties. We
have expressed the topic of this essay as question: In what sense, if any,
can the modern physician consistently be, in creed, a loyalist? Thus, I am
writing not so much about professional medical ethics as a whole, but
about the ethics of physicians. Nevertheless, I think most of what I say
about physicians applies to nurses as well. Also, I think physicians, taken
as a whole, stand to benefit greatly by examining the virtues of their sibling profession. I hold (though my argument will have to be deferred) that
the nursing profession has, by and large, been truer to the spirit of loyalty
than have physicians. A third area of bias is my concern with the physician primarily as clinician, to the neglect of several important issues that
concern researchers. This limitation is imposed, for the most part, to contain the length of the essay.

A comprehensive treatment of medical ethics would also include a
development of the role and responsibilities of patients. This topic will be
treated only briefly in this essay. Once again, I am interested in developing a professional ethics for physicians. This task, as we have discussed, is
not solely a matter of formulating the "goods internal to a practice." A
professional ethic of loyalty is something public, aiming at and articulat-
ing not only the special features of medicine that ought to endear it to its
practitioners, but also goods that apply to everyone involved in health
care. Thus, patients will play a central role in our discussion, and their
views will always be relevant. Specifically, though, we will be interested in
their views about physicians.

I should comment about the use of unpublished material by Royce.
As several Royce scholars have pointed out, it is difficult to treat Royce's
ethics fairly without consulting his unpublished works. In this essay, I
make use of his early Lectures in the History of Ethics, his middle Pittsburgh Lectures and his later Extension Course in Ethics. My references to
the Pittsburgh Lectures are considerably more detailed than any previous

author's, consonant with my general emphasis on Royce's middle period, in which he addressed himself most explicitly to the type of identity problems—personal and tradition bound—constituting the formal problem of this essay. This use of the Pittsburgh Lectures is both a blessing and a handicap. On the negative side, the inquisitive reader is hampered by the difficulty of referring back to the referenced text. On the positive side, Royce scholars will be treated to new material.

There is one final preliminary that I believe will be worthwhile—a look at the thought of Alasdair MacIntyre.

ROYCE AND MACINTYRE

Persons familiar with the philosophy of Alasdair MacIntyre will detect in Royce many of MacIntyre's concerns and convictions. Indeed, the similarities between the thinkers are so extensive that the charge of redundancy might be leveled at the present work because it contains material that MacIntyre has already recognized and articulated. To address this criticism, I will first consider some specific views shared by both MacIntyre and Royce. We will find, I believe, that Royce and MacIntyre cover similar material in a complementary, rather than overlapping, manner. Furthermore, differences between the two thinkers certainly do exist, and a couple of these will be highlighted. This topic warrants a brief detour not only because the relationship between the two approaches must be clarified but also because MacIntyre may serve as a useful orienting device to those who are unfamiliar with Royce.

I would like to call attention to four similarities between MacIntyre and Royce that are relevant to my project: (1) they employ a similar historico-philosophical method, embodying similar views about the mission and status of philosophy; (2) they offer an account of the virtues, including a unifying virtue, which intertwines the notion of selfhood with the notion of community; (3) they both adhere to a nondogmatic, fallibilistic form of absolutism; and (4) they both may be considered, in certain crucial respects, to be pragmatists, while diverging in similar ways from classical American pragmatism as it is developed in the writings of Dewey and James.

MacIntyre often refers to himself as a philosophical historian and cites Hegel and Collingwood as colleagues in this enterprise (AV, 3–4).

Were he a more avid student of the American tradition, he would certainly also include Royce. Several key elements in the historical labor of MacIntyre and Royce coincide. Both thinkers acknowledge that the only valid kind of history is one that is self-consciously informed by standards; historical inquiry is always an expression of the values and purposes of the inquirers. Both would warn against treating historical figures "as contributors to a single debate with a relatively unvarying subject matter" (AV, 11). As historicists, MacIntyre and Royce want to appropriate the works of early philosophers for their present purposes. But they are careful not to project these purposes, at least in the modern form, retrogradely into the antecedent historical milieu.

This point is best understood as the result of another important similarity. Both MacIntyre and Royce hold that it is impossible to understand problems in philosophy as anything other than the culmination of historical processes (AV, 269; SMP, 9). We cannot, in their view, thoroughly abstract a thinker from his sociocultural milieu; and we cannot understand sociocultural milieus, and their characteristic issues, in anything but historical terms. Thus, Richard Cabot wrote of Royce, "No other teacher of philosophy in my time has carried into his seminars so full and living a consciousness of the historic stream of philosophic thought" (1916, 468). For philosophical historians such as MacIntyre and Royce, the questions that occupy modern philosophers are unique, but unique only because they arise at a certain moment in the history of thought. These questions can and should be traced to historical antecedents. Their present form, however, cannot be foisted back upon philosophical forefathers. History travels forward, not backward.

MacIntyre and Royce identify the stimuli to philosophical inquiries as historically contingent problem situations (MacIntyre 1988, 355; PC, 361). MacIntyre begins *After Virtue* by illustrating the interminable nature of present moral debates, and the rest of that book consists essentially of an elaborate and masterly historical-philosophical account of the nature of this problem. *After Virtue* becomes one of the finest examples available of what Dewey referred to as "the circumscription of a problem situation." In *The Philosophy of Loyalty* Royce begins with a similar problem—the effect of the absence of coherent moral foundations on current scientific, spiritual, and social life—and, as with MacIntyre, immediately observes that the enfeeblement of moral foundations is largely the result of a modern disregard for traditions. Though Royce (and, again, MacIntyre) agrees that our traditions must be revised, he opposes the modern propensity for presenting moral alternatives as if they existed in a historical vacuum. In this vein, Royce writes:

> Moreover, since moral standards, as Antigone said, are not of today or yesterday, I believe that revision does not mean, in this field, a mere break with the past. I myself have spent my life in revising my opinions. And yet, whenever I have most carefully revised my moral standards, I am always able to see, upon reviewing my course of thought that at best I have been finding out, in some new light, the true meaning that was latent in old traditions. Those traditions were often better in spirit than the fathers knew. (PL, 7)

Our comparison of MacIntyre and Royce has, I believe, already yielded two good reasons for studying Royce. First, the notion that moral life is vitiated by the disjunction of moral principles and moral traditions occurred to Royce before it occurred to MacIntyre, just as it occurred, in another form, in the context of quite different concerns, to Augustine and Hegel before Royce. And, just as Royce, Peirce, Dewey, and others in the American tradition drew both consciously and unconsciously from Augustine and Hegel, MacIntyre inherits the legacy of these American thinkers, especially Royce, whether he acknowledges it or not. If MacIntyre is to be consistent with his own premises, he must understand the family history of his central thesis.

Second, Royce's remark that the ideas expressed in a tradition are often more potent than the forefathers knew is related to one of his central metaphysical theses, the claim that human judgments—whether they be moral, prudential, epistemic, or aesthetic—embody a teleological impulse ultimately fulfilled only in a comprehensive unity of human actions and intentions. This impulse is often latent and tends to express itself in seemingly inexplicable aspects of theories and, of course, in the form of differing and incompatible traditions. Royce, in offering a comprehensive metaphysical justification of this thesis, provides substantial groundwork for a conception of philosophical history similar to MacIntyre's.

Part and parcel of the notion that inquiry begins with a historically contingent problem situation is the belief that traditions are sustained by conflicts. MacIntyre writes, "A living tradition then is an historically extended, socially embodied argument and an argument precisely in part about the goods which constitute that tradition" (AV, 222). MacIntyre contributes substantially to our understanding of this point through his discussion of the tragic protagonist, who grapples with incompatible alternatives engendered within a moral tradition. MacIntyre rightly points out that the alternatives presented to the tragic protagonist, occurring as they do within the context of a single tradition, differ from those arising from the counterposition of incommensurable moral outlooks. Also notable in MacIntyre's discussion is the prescription that the tragic protagonist be evaluated in terms of his exhibition of virtue, rather than by his choice between alternatives (AV, 224). MacIntyre here makes the same point that Royce makes in his discussion of Robert E. Lee (PL, 90–91): that, within the context of a single scheme of moral life, ambiguities and alternatives will inevitably arise and that persons should be judged by the integrity with which they respond to these situations, rather than by the ultimate verdict concerning the rightness of their choices.

Nevertheless, what MacIntyre recognizes but does not develop as fully as Royce is the idea that the conflicts that sustain traditions consist of series of interpretations and counter-interpretations of the ideals of communities. That is, Royce, more than MacIntyre, details how the goods constituting a tradition are the ideals that define a community. Once again, Royce's account of the relation between a community and its ideals is developed in the context of his theory of interpretation. Were MacIntyre to attend to this account, I think his thought would be enriched.

Another problem with which Royce can be helpful is the problem of what occurs, and what should be done, when traditions collide. On such occasions, criteria for evaluating the conflicting traditions must be developed. Three characteristics of such criteria are certain: (1) they will not be impartial, (2) they will be transformative, and (3) they will effect a transformation in the direction of impartiality. Their non-impartiality consists in the fact that they must issue from the competing traditions and will hence reflect the outlook of those traditions. They will be transformative because they will have an effect on the traditions from which they arise. These transformations will aim in the direction of inter-traditional impartiality because they will accord priority to values that emerge out of both traditions. Royce offers a criterion—the criterion of loyalty to the great community—designed to manifest these characteristics while medi-

ating the conflicts between several traditions. To understand Royce's justification of the principle of loyalty to the great community, in its fullest
form, would require comprehensive study. The reader may expect only a
fragment of such a project within the confines of this essay.

We are now ready to move on to the second general area of agreement
between MacIntyre and Royce—they offer accounts of the virtues, including a unifying virtue, that intertwine the notions of selfhood and
community. MacIntyre describes three stages in an adequate account of
the virtues. First, one must describe how virtues are conceived within the
framework of practices. MacIntyre's notion of a practice (AV, 187) is rich
and useful, and it has no well-defined correlate within the work of Royce.
Practices are constituted by the cooperative activities of certain types of
dynamic communities, such as a community of health-care providers. At
this stage of the account, virtues are conceived roughly as excellences relevant to the ideals characterizing a practice. The attainment of virtue becomes, from this perspective, a good that is internal to the practice. At the
second stage, an account of virtue is given that aligns it with the movement toward the good for humans. A practice-specific notion of virtue
thus gives way to a species-specific notion. The existence of a human *telos*
is hypothesized, and virtue is described in terms of the movement toward
this goal. In the final stage, the *telos* is fleshed out by examining its relation to a moral tradition. The quest for an ultimate human good becomes
a community project.

Royce offers an account of loyalty that evolves through each of these
stages. Royce's discussion of loyalty begins in the context of what he calls
"natural communities." For now, it will be enough to say that practices and
natural communities are related by the fact that the former develop only
in the context of the latter. The need emerges to justify loyalty in terms different from a seemingly arbitrary appeal to the interests of natural communities, and Royce develops the notion of loyalty to loyalty, which is an
expression for loyalty justified by a certain kind of universal human *telos*.
Finally, Royce fleshes out the account of loyalty to loyalty with a theological account of the characteristics of a great or beloved community,
grounding the *telos* with an appeal to Christianity and its tradition.

At every stage of development, Royce's account tends to complement
and enrich MacIntyre's. A significant convergence is reflected in the following passage from MacIntyre:

I have suggested so far that unless there is a *telos* which transcends the limited goods of practices by constituting the good of a whole human life, the good of a human life conceived as a unity, it will *both* be the case that a certain subversive arbitrariness will invade the moral life *and* that we shall be unable to specify the context of certain virtues adequately. These two considerations are reinforced by a third: that there is at least one virtue recognized by the tradition which cannot be specified at all except with reference to the wholeness of human life—the virtue of integrity or constancy. . . . This notion of singleness of purpose in a whole life can have no application unless that of a whole life does. (AV, 203)[4]

If we substitute the term *natural communities* for "practices," and *loyalty* for "integrity," this quote would be a wholly adequate statement of Royce's position. This observation is of no small moment—it seems that both Royce and MacIntyre have specified a unifying virtue, and, though they call it by different names, it is in each case the same virtue. Royce, however, gives a much fuller account of this virtue than MacIntyre.

Both Royce and MacIntyre treat the virtues in accounts grounded in a notion of selfhood which holds that: (1) the self is informed by sociocultural standards (AV, 33, 59, 104); (2) the self is expanded through a social vision founded on community membership (AV, 34, 202); (3) selfhood is unintelligible outside of a context that includes plans or goals (AV, 34, 205, 215); and (4) the identity crisis is a nearly unavoidable aspect of the development of a modern self (citations confined to MacIntyre since Royce's positons on these matters will be discussed at length in this study). The latter thesis is not specifically discussed by MacIntyre in *After Virtue*, but it follows from his analysis. In fact, both thinkers begin the study of the self with the same fundamental question: In what does the unity of an individual life consist? The two thinkers, I believe, give similar answers. MacIntyre spends much of his time in *After Virtue* showing that alternative accounts are conceptually inadequate; Royce tackles the same project in *The World and the Individual*. However, in *The Philosophy of Loyalty*, and in several of his lectures between 1907 and 1910, Royce also tries to show that alternative accounts of the unity of a self are *psychologically* inadequate, something that MacIntyre has never attempted. It is this latter line of reasoning that we will be tracing in this essay, and so, once again, we find ourselves covering matters that are not at all redundant but that complement and enrich what we find in MacIntyre. MacIntyre presents the problems of modern moral philosophy as stemming from an epistemological crisis. Royce would in many respects agree with MacIntyre's analysis. But Royce adds that the epistemological crisis is attended by a psychological crisis, that the two are inseparable, and that we must attend to both.

The third major similarity—adherence to a nondogmatic, fallibilistic form of absolutism—is important, but I will discuss it here only by noting that this aspect of both thinkers is the vantage point from which they criticize Hegel. MacIntyre writes in *Whose Justice? Which Rationality?*:

> Yet if in what it moves from, tradition-constituted enquiry is anti-Cartesian, in what it moves toward, tradition-constituted enquiry is anti-Hegelian. Implicit in the rationality of such enquiry there is indeed a conception of a final truth, that is to say, a relationship of the mind to its objects which would be wholly adequate in respect of the capacities of that mind. But any conception of that state as one in which the mind could by its own powers know itself as thus adequately informed is ruled out; the Absolute Knowledge of the Hegelian system is from this tradition-constituted standpoint a chimaera. No one at any stage can ever rule out the future possibility of their present beliefs and judgments being shown to be inadequate in a variety of ways. (361)

Royce, as Oppenheim points out (1993, 200–201), would agree.[5]

Regarding the fourth point—a similar theoretical relation to American pragmatism—the case for viewing Royce as a pragmatist, on the one hand, has already been substantially made by Mahowald, and her arguments should be enriched by much of what we cover in this essay. The notion that MacIntyre is in certain respects similar to a pragmatist, on the other hand, has been suggested but not defended (Porter 1993, 536). I would like to point the way toward such a defense with a few observations. First, as we discussed earlier, MacIntyre views philosophy as a problem-oriented enterprise, and this view, most certainly, is a characteristic of

classical American pragmatism. Second, MacIntyre, with Peirce, is a fallibilist, while also holding that some beliefs cannot, from a given historical
perspective, be doubted. Third, MacIntyre, with all the pragmatists, holds
that theory and action are ineradicably united, and that all thought is purposive (AV, 61). And fourth, related to the previous consideration, Mac-
Intyre stresses that "facts" or "perceptions" are never independent but are
always funded by previous facts, perceptions, and theorizations (AV,
79–80). Royce, once again, agrees on each of these points. Further, Mac-
Intyre's critique of perspectivism in *Whose Justice? Which Rationality?*
(351ff.) corresponds in many ways to Royce's critique of Jamesian and
Deweyan pragmatism, particularly in his insistence that perspectivist critiques of absolutism are based on an inadequate understanding of the
conceptual importance of the absolutist notion of truth (367).

There are, of course, topics of disagreement between MacIntyre and
Royce. One of the most obvious is that Royce is a metaphysical idealist,
MacIntyre is not.[6] This disagreement will not be highly important with regard to the mission of this essay. Here Royce's ethical idealism will be defended on the basis of a pragmatic argument that does not depend, at least
in any simple or direct manner, on the truth of metaphysical idealism.

I would like to call attention to two areas of divergence that may be
more important to our project. Each of these is no doubt related to some
degree to more basic metaphysical differences, but such relations will, for
the present, remain subterranean. The first is with regard to the thinkers'
respective estimation of Enlightenment philosophy. Both present similar
criticisms. But whereas MacIntyre writes as if the Enlightenment project
was at best a detour, at worst a total dead end, Royce conceives Enlightenment failures more as profitable lessons, as advances. I submit that
MacIntyre's line of argument goes somewhat astray. MacIntyre lays such
great emphasis on the destructiveness of the Enlightenment's belief in the
fixity of subject matter of ethics (1990, 28; AV, 11) that he neglects to recognize how the subject matter of ethics is, by the tenets of his own theory, indeed fixed. This point may best be illustrated by referring to an argument from *Three Rival Versions of Moral Enquiry*:

> So we are threatened by an apparent paradox in the understand-
> ing of moral enquiry as a type of craft: only insofar as we have
> already arrived at certain conclusions are we able to become the

sort of person able to engage in such enquiry so as to reach sound conclusions. How is this threat of paradox—recognizably a version of that posed at the outset by Plato in the *Meno* about learning in general—to be circumvented, dissolved, or otherwise met? The answer is in part that suggested by the *Meno*: unless we already have within ourselves the potentiality for moving towards and achieving the relevant theoretical and practical conclusions we shall be unable to learn. But we also need a teacher to enable us to actualize that potentiality, and we shall have to learn from that teacher and initially accept on the basis of his or her authority within the community of a craft precisely what intellectual and moral habits it is which we must cultivate and acquire if we are to become effective self-moved participants in such enquiry. (63)

Since MacIntyre acknowledges both that the true good is fixed and absolute (1990, 59–60; 66) and that individuals, even prior to their exposure to a tradition, are specially suited to the pursuit of this good, it seems to follow that the subject matter of ethics will indeed be fixed to a certain degree, notwithstanding that different ages will have varying ways of approaching and conceptualizing it.

There are, in the above passage, two parts to MacIntyre's solution to the paradox of how moral inquiry may commence: (1) we have something within or about ourselves that makes us fit for this inquiry (in Plato's case, our innate ideas); and (2) we recognize authority. MacIntyre goes on to stress the second of these aspects, to the neglect of the first. In so doing, I believe Royce would say that MacIntyre fails to recognize the contribution of Enlightenment thinkers to our understanding how the individual is fit for moral inquiry. Descartes' theory of innate ideas, or Kant's account of the contribution of the mind to experience, are examples. It is certainly the case that the Enlightenment was overly impressed with the individual. Nevertheless, it is also the case that the scholastics were overly impressed with authority. For Royce, we are able to learn from the successes and failures of both movements.

Perhaps MacIntyre would have done better to focus more on the Enlightenment tendency to view the history of thought as a relentless progression toward perfection.[7] This attitude—with the attendant faith that when something good develops it will be preserved—is no doubt centrally related to the propensity of Enlightenment thinkers to disregard the wisdom of the past. Royce's rejection of the meliorism common in the Enlightenment (most evident in his critiques of Spencer) is shared by MacIntyre and is another factor that separates the thinkers from the likes of Dewey or de Chardin.[8]

A second area of divergence between MacIntyre and Royce is with regard to the complexity and variety of fundamental choices that each thinker views as being available to moral agents. Royce, on the one hand, is impressed with the diversity of legitimate theoretical alternatives that present themselves to budding moral agents. Further, Royce finds this pluralism of opportunities to be a generally welcome result of developments spurred by the Enlightenment. MacIntyre, on the other hand, tends to emphasize, somewhat more than Royce, the importance of what is inherited from the past and how it limits our ability to adjust ourselves to alternative outlooks.[9] Whereas MacIntyre frequently stresses the fact that rationality is conceivable only within a tradition and that various traditions will engender largely irreconcilable notions of rationality, Royce would note that many moral traditions, emerging as they do from various communities, share similar notions of rationality. Stated otherwise, Royce's point is that a multitude of moral traditions may evolve within the framework of a single relatively uniform intellectual tradition, with a single relatively uniform understanding of rationality. In witness to this claim, Royce might cite the plurality of moral theories that are represented, by MacIntyre's count, within the Enlightenment tradition. Further, Royce would want to reemphasize a point of MacIntyre's: that irreconcilable traditions are not necessarily incommensurable, that often there is enough common ground that we can fruitfully compare and contrast views that emerge even from conflicting accounts of rationality. In this spirit, Royce would no doubt want to point out that MacIntyre is himself a product of the Enlightenment, that his brand of Thomism has benefited in numerous ways from his exposure to thinkers such as Descartes, Kant, and even Sidgwick, and, in fact, that MacIntyre could never have written *After Virtue* or developed the theory of rationality contained in *Whose Justice? Which Rationality?* without the benefit of his Enlightenment ancestors.

Certainly the difference here indicated between Royce and MacIntyre is only one of degree. MacIntyre acknowledges that the search for a human good must lead us beyond the bounds of family, neighborhood, city, or tribe (AV, 221). He not only believes it is possible to situate oneself within the context of rival traditions (not simultaneously, but consecutively), but precisely that is one of his stated objectives in *Three Rival Versions of Moral Enquiry* (43). Likewise, Royce, as we have seen, acknowledges the ineradicable influence—mediated through tradition, culture, and other forms of human interaction—of our historically contingent memberships within given communities.

ADVICE TO READERS

In the introduction, I have outlined the orientation and purpose of our inquiry and sketched the basic, Roycean movement of thought that I hope will lead us from our current dissatisfaction with medicine and its moral tradition to a better, more promising future. Also, I have compared and contrasted Royce with a prominent contemporary thinker, hoping to make Royce more accessible to readers who are not grounded in classical American philosophy.

One more task remains. In anticipation of a readership that includes some persons who are not trained in philosophy, I would like to suggest a strategy for circumventing some of the more technically difficult sections of the book. I believe it is possible for such persons to read selectively, without missing out on the major theses of the book. To this end, I will conclude with a brief synopsis of each chapter together with guidance about how the chapter might be approached by more casual readers, including undergraduate students and health-care professionals.

Chapter 1 should be read in its entirety. It is here that we delineate the problems of medicine and its tradition that set the stage for the rest of our inquiry. Apart from this chapter, the rest of the book would lose focus. Further, the discussion here is rather untechnical and should not be problematic for most readers.

Chapter 2 delves into Royce's account of the development of personal identity and contains some matters that the casual reader will find challenging. This is particularly true of the section "Royce on Imitation." However, the sections entitled "Opposition, Crisis and the Birth of the Self" and "The Paradoxical Nature of Idealization" are necessary to the movement of thought in the essay. Though they are rather technical in places, they are not as challenging as "Royce on Imitation" and will reward the attention of both of the specialist and nonspecialist. The final section, "Three Ideals of Personality," is essential but is less technical than the rest of the chapter. The hurried student might want to confine the initial reading of chapter 2 to this final section, but some later filling in would be necessary.

Chapter 3 is dedicated to characterizing the Roycean doctrine and art of loyalty. The section entitled "Community and Interpretation" is quite technical and is provided primarily for the trained philosopher, though I believe it will reward the general reader who seeks a deeper understanding of the text.

In chapter 4, I seek to provide philosophical and psychological support for Royce's doctrine of loyalty. Philosophically speaking, this chapter is perhaps the most important part of the book. It is here that Royce's doctrine receives its primary structural support. As we cover Royce's moral insight, and compare it with the insights of other philosophers, the reader should come to a much deeper understanding of Royce. Further, appreciating the value of Royce's theory, even for nontheoretical purposes, would be difficult for one who has not studied this chapter.

Chapters 5, 6, and 7 are where we use Royce's theory to tackle the problems that we developed in the first chapter. Each chapter should be read, more or less, in its entirety. Though there are technically difficult passages, each section contains material that should be interesting to a broad readership.

Finally, Chapter 8, in which the art of loyalty is approached in its capacity as a living option for individual physicians, is less technical than the others and should not be difficult.

It is my hope that this book can serve in some way to vitalize the spirit of interpretation that Royce recognized to be the guiding force of every genuine community. I seek not so much to persuade as to stimulate thought and discussion. My aim is to engage thinkers with non-Roycean perspectives in a common, humanitarian undertaking and not merely to refute them. Such engagement, I believe, fosters the fellowship that characterizes all genuine inquiry.

1

❖

Medicine's Fractured
Tradition

As a premed student in the 1970s I often heard of the "Marcus Welby complex." According to medical school admissions committees, there were legions of aspiring doctors with a naive vision of medical heroism, exemplified by Robert Young's television character, Marcus Welby. As most viewers probably remember, Welby was knowledgeable, insightful, confident, understanding and compassionate. He was a model of competence, rewarded by a happy life, the gratitude of his patients, high standing in the community, and, presumably, a profound sense of fulfillment.

The feeling among committee members was that individuals who aspired to Welbyism would be bitterly disappointed, discouraged, and alienated when they became acquainted with the real world of medicine, where patients were rarely grateful, saving lives was less than commonplace, and where ideals tended to become frayed around the edges. Just what the committees wanted was not so clear, at least to me; but they seemed unanimous in eschewing utopian ideals of medicine. If there was no obvious positive advice, there was still the negative injunction—"Medicine is not perfect. Do not expect the world to be laid out at your feet."

The purveyors of such negative wisdom probably drew more from their personal experience as physicians than they did from observing the careers of student doctors. Indeed, the majority of these senior administrators probably began their own careers as Welbyan idealists, an outlook that is only natural for beginners. What the committee members learned is that Welbyism is impractical. And they had the vision to see that it was becoming more impractical all the time.

In this chapter I will explore some of the reasons why the ideal exemplified by heroes such as Marcus Welby has become obsolete. I will discuss the dominant tradition in medicine—what I will call, with Jonsen, the "ethics of competence"—and show how this tradition once engendered a Welbyan sort of ideal. I will argue that recent developments in the field of medicine have exposed fundamental inconsistencies that plague the tradition, weakening the old ideal and demanding its further revision.

This chapter can be viewed essentially as the circumscription of a problem. With this in mind, I will begin by illustrating what I call a "double bind" problem in medicine.

THE DOUBLE BIND

Let us consider the circumstances of a modern emergency department (ED) physician. Today's young ED physician may have as much in common with tomorrow's schizophrenic as with Marcus Welby. Both the ED physician and the schizophrenic are apt to experience what has been described by developmental psychologists as a "double bind" situation. The double bind occurs when a person is dedicated to an ideal that cannot be achieved because it requires incompatible alternatives (Bateson et al., 1956). For example, a young boy may be dedicated to pleasing his mother. But if his mother asks him to insulate the attic and also expects him to stay clean and neat at all times, the child is confronted with mutually exclusive imperatives: (1) insulate the attic and (2) stay clean and neat. If he does the job, he will get dirty; he will be chastised by his mother for disorderliness, and he will fail to achieve his ideal of pleasing Mom. If he refrains from doing the job, and concentrates on staying clean, he will be scolded for laziness and once again will fail to achieve his ideal. The boy is doomed to failure from the outset. Because this ideal is so central for the youngster, his self-image is apt to be shattered by repeated failures. Possibly he will retreat into a dream world where it is possible to perform all manner of dirty jobs while maintaining perfect decorum. Whatever the avenue, the child is likely to break away from the proverbial "real world."

The modern ED physician tends also to have a central ideal: "Practice according to the standard of care."[1] And, just like the young schizophrenic, the physician's ideal often imposes contradictory imperatives.

Suppose our physician is taking care of a five-year-old who tripped while chasing his sister and hit his head on a coffee table. According to his mother, the child had a brief—less than a minute—loss of consciousness. He also vomited twice just after regaining consciousness. Since then, the child has done well. He has been active and alert and suffers no amnesia. On exam, the child has a sizable contusion on his forehead; his mental status is normal and there are no neurological deficits. Our ED physician wants to apply the golden rule—"Practice according to the standard of care"—but faces a quandary. The standard of care in such situations varies according to the particular authority one consults. Several authors would recommend a CT scan (Dietrich et al. 1993; Stein and Ross 1993; Harad and Kerstein 1992; Shackford et al. 1992); others would not (Mohanty, Thompson, and Rakower 1991; Rimel and Jane 1985; Duus et al. 1994).

Examination of a multitude of relevant journal articles reveals not only that the risk of significant intracranial injury in such cases is not well established (despite extensive study) but that, even when there are compatible data, risk-benefit analyses tend to vary. For example, Dietrich et al. noted a 5 percent incidence of intracranial pathology in neurologically intact children with head injuries; and in a sample of older head-injured patients who were also neurologically stable, Mohanty, Thompson, and Rakower discovered a similar 3.5 percent incidence of intracranial pathology. But, whereas Dietrich's group took this statistic as good evidence that patients with minor head injuries should be scanned, Mohanty and colleagues drew the opposite conclusion. The Dietrich group pointed to the fact that persons with intracranial pathology, even if they do not require surgical intervention (they did not specify which, if any, of their patients needed surgery), run a high risk for developing negative sequelae and therefore ought to be singled out for closer follow-up. Mohanty's group, on the other hand, noted that none of twelve neurologically stable patients in their study who had positive CT scans needed surgical intervention and pointed out that no untoward sequelae would result from the decision not to scan (presumably because conditions such as postconcussive syndrome are not preventable by therapeutic interventions).

In days of old, it would have been simple for our physician to decide that, because the usefulness of the given intervention is not clearly determined, it is better to err on the side of thoroughness and, therefore, order the scan. Perhaps if we are to understand *standard of care* strictly in terms of the avoidance of negligence, this decision would be consonant with our ED physician's stated ideal. On the other hand, the standard of care may no longer fit so nicely within its traditional locus in tort law. George Annas writes:

> 'Standard of care' is a legal term denoting the level of conduct a physician or health care provider must meet in treating a patient so as not to be guilty of negligence, usually called malpractice. That standard is generally defined simply as what a reasonably prudent physician (or specialist) would do in the same or similar circumstances. (1993, 4)

But if we are to identify *standard of care* with the "reasonably prudent physician" standard, it seems we must look beyond the courtroom. For medicine in the 1990s, prudence involves more than shrewdness in avoiding lawsuits. It also necessitates an eye toward cost containment, which, even more than legal acumen, is becoming a matter of survival for practicing physicians. For the purposes of an ordinary ED physician in this country, *standard of care* is understood in the broader context; it is the standard of prudence regarding legal, financial, and institutional aspects of medical practice.

The situation, then, is this: The ED physician who orders the CT scan will fail to practice according to the standard of care, at least as the standard is understood by certain colleagues—by most radiologists (who prefer to minimize unscheduled scans) and by others who are concerned to control the costs of medical care; the physician who does not order the scan will fail to meet the standard of care as it is understood by still other colleagues and by any lawyer who might want to show the physician liable if the child subsequently develops neuropsychological problems, such as a motor deficit or the failure to advance in first-grade reading classes. No matter what the decision, the physician will fail to practice according to the standard of care. No matter which strategy is employed, the physician will likely suffer condemnation from some quarter for lacking sound clinical judgment—perhaps, on one hand, from insurance organizations, hospital administrators, and politicians because of indiscriminate spending; on the other hand, from patients and from the law for exposing patients to risk.

The dilemma of ED physicians is replayed throughout the world of medicine wherever physicians or other care providers must face the contradictory demands of providing cutting-edge-quality care and minimizing cost. Consider TennCare, Tennessee's new health care plan, which is instituting capitated contracts in order to force physicians, by threat of financial loss, to spend less. At the same time, Tennessee physicians remain liable for bad outcomes. Thus, society entreats physicians to avoid expensive clinical investigations aimed at uncovering unlikely diseases but also prosecutes them for failing to undertake these same clinical investigations—whenever it turns out that the unlikely diseases were actually present.[2] Only a clairvoyant could operate successfully under these conditions. TennCare's and similar policies are, within the context of our present medicolegal situation, contradictions. And clinical guidelines are generally not helpful—as we have seen in the case of CT scans for pediatric head trauma—because different guidelines will reflect incompatible poles of the contradictory general standard.

More than risk-benefit polarity undermines attempts to meet the standard of care. Medicine is increasingly recognized as a customer service profession. If the standard of care is to be met, the physician must make all reasonable attempts to satisfy the patient (Schoeneweis 1992, 1). The customer-service imperative becomes problematic when one considers that patients frequently desire more testing, more prescribing, and more specialty evaluation—more care—than general standards within the medical profession would indicate.[3] The double bind is apt to occur when a patient demands care that will likely be condemned by most (but not all) reviewers. The physician in this situation will inevitably be assaulted by one flank or the other. If acquiescing to the patient's wishes, the physician will be accused of wasting medical resources, exposing the patient to unnecessary risks, and/or perpetuating unsubstantiated, unscientific clinical practices. To go against the patient's wishes and to opt for prudent, scientifically substantiated strategies means that the physician will be accused of disregarding the patient's special needs.

In ED medicine, and in other forms of primary care, another common double bind occurs in situations where specialty consultation has been enlisted. Occasionally, the ED physician will receive advice from a specialist that contradicts the referring physician's medical judgment. Now it is generally believed within the ranks of physicians, laymen, and the judiciary that a consultant's opinion is more authoritative than a consulter's. However, any ED physician is ultimately held responsible for whatever lies within that physician's clinical purview. For instance, a recent case study in *Foresight*, a risk management newsletter published by the American College of Emergency Physicians, details the situation of an emergency physician who has a patient with lower abdominal pain, whom he believes has a risk, albeit low, of having an ectopic pregnancy. He wants to admit the patient, but his gynecology consultant advises him to discharge her, citing the low likelihood of a serious problem. *Foresight* makes the point that the ED physician will be held accountable if he discharges his patient. If she goes on to develop serious consequences, he will be blamed, since he had reason to believe she was at risk (Howell et al. 1994, 4). The problem (not addressed in *Foresight*) is this: Unless that ED physician can produce an overwhelming argument that (1) refutes his consultant's claims or (2) demonstrates that the management decision was clearly beyond the reasonable scope of competent ED physicians, he is once again apt to wind up outside the standard of care. If he insists on inpatient management, he has forsaken the normal source of guidance and opted for a more expensive alternative. To carry this off he must be able to explain himself to all concerned—often to health care bureaucrats who rely on expert testimony to form their medical opinions. But in the eyes of at least one so-called expert, he will be in conflict with the elusive standard.

Even if we restrict our concerns about the standard of care to matters of legal negligence, the modern ED physician is subject to double binds. Falk and Cohn tell the story of an emergency physician who practices in a facility that lacks a CT scanner but who has a patient needing a CT scan:

> The magnitude of his dilemma approaches the asymptote of insolubility, for he must somehow weigh the risks and delays of transporting the patient against the alternatives available in-house. Unfortunately, he must do so at his peril, for if the consequences to the patient are adverse, he can be assured he will inevitably face Monday morning quarterbacking as he views the ensuing malpractice imbroglio from his box seat in the dock. . . .
>
> Whatever the attending physician's decision, he must make it quickly, even instinctively, for every second may be precious.

Any factor he overlooks may return to haunt him in the form of second-guessing in a malpractice suit. So there must he sit, out on a limb fashioned by hands not his own, naked in his solitude, his reputation hanging not on his honest judgment or good faith best efforts, but on success or failure, plain and simple. (1982, 218–219)

On many occasions similar to the one noted above, poor outcomes will eventuate no matter what options those attending employ. Once again, we have double binds.

Of course, all professions have controversies. But a double bind is no mere controversy. It is a dilemma that cannot be resolved without a major overhaul of the identity of the subject. The child who faces recurrent double binds will eventually take on two separate identities. Most physicians view themselves as knowledgeable, thorough, frugal, and compassionate. These qualities represent more than mere professional strategies. They are viewed as elements of character by the physician, components of his personal, or at least professional, identity. But when being frugal repeatedly causes him to fail at being thorough, or when acting knowledgeably leads to recurrent questions about his compassion, his identity as a physician is assaulted. Analogous to the self-understanding of a schizophrenic, the professional self-understanding of a physician must then undergo radical reorganization. If he cannot be both frugal and thorough, knowledgeable and compassionate, then he must find a new guiding standard. But we are ahead of the game. Before we can discuss new standards, we must go into more detail about the old.

THE ETHICS OF COMPETENCE

We have identified a double bind problem in clinical medicine, and we have indicated that this problem is related to medicine's axiom— "Practice according to the standard of care"—which is often interpreted in contradictory ways. When viewed as a fundamental statement of the aims of practitioners, as the axiom often is, yet another shortcoming becomes apparent—the axiom's incompleteness. Specifically, there is nothing in the principle that helps a physician cope with the brutality of life on the wards or in the ED. It possesses no motivating power. It does not help the physician solve the riddle of how to live serenely amidst violence and suffering. It leaves him with pressing questions: Why should he regularly submit to the foul language, the smell of urine, and the torrents of emesis that occasion the care of belligerent and intoxicated patients? How can he maintain a positive outlook after telling weeping parents there was nothing he could do for their child? For what purpose should he give up his social life or endure long hours of sleeplessness? In order to meet the standard of care, the physician will often be called upon to make great sacrifices. But where is the justification for this sacrifice? Some would argue that justification lies in the considerable remuneration and prestige that accompanies the practice of medicine. But there are certainly easier ways to make money or garner prestige. Further, such a reply begets another question: Why should the practice of medicine pay so highly or command such respect? To answer these questions, we must turn to the tradition that nurtures and transcends medicine's guiding maxim.

The most recent form of the grand tradition in medicine is probably best understood in terms of what Jonsen has identified as an "ethics of competence," exemplified in the teachings of Josiah Royce's student, colleague, and friend at Harvard, Richard Cabot. The ethics of competence is an extension of the Hippocratic tradition, together with elements of Judeo-Christian humanitarianism. Jonsen writes:

> The ethics of competence, fully understood as mastery of the science and skills of diagnosis, therapy and prevention of disease, together with an appreciation of the personal and social aspects of the patient's health and disease, are the glory of modern medicine. They are the standard to which all physicians must be held—the goal of medical education and the expectation of the public. These ethics of competence might well be given the eponym "Cabotean ethics," since Dr. Cabot did so much to articulate them. They can stand as the modern extension of Hippocratic ethics into the age of scientific medicine. (Jonsen 1990, 27)

The ethics of competence, and the tradition it represents, is no mere set of rules for the morally acceptable behavior of physicians. It is an ideal and a momentum generated out of centuries of medical practice.

Through this ideal the physician defines himself—his role, his standing, his professional cause—and is understood by society. This medical tradition has more than historical significance; it is a dynamic modern force. Apart from such a tradition, the concept of a medical community would be incoherent (as we shall later see in detail). The tradition shapes the future of medicine even as it is affected by tendencies and incidents occurring outside its realm of influence. Neither the current explosion of medical technologies nor the recognition of their significance are possible apart from the perspective of this medical tradition. Surely students would balk before the rigors of modern medical education if not enticed by the image of what it means to be a physician—an image projected through the lens of medicine's grand tradition.

To practice according to the standard of care, then, may be the ruling maxim for some of medicine's practitioners, but it is not their *raison d'être*. It is a central maxim appearing as medicine's tradition has evolved. The standard-of-care maxim is justified by this tradition, and it can be correctly understood only in the context of this tradition. Jonsen and others have chronicled the development of medicine's grand tradition, and we will not replicate such an undertaking here. It will be helpful, however, to review a few of its central, problematic aspects.

The origins of Western medicine are often traced to the teachings of Hippocrates of Cos and his followers. Though there are few historical details of the life of Hippocrates, texts written by his disciples (which for many years were erroneously attributed to Hippocrates himself) provide a substantial basis for understanding the Hippocratic tradition.

This tradition has, at times, been portrayed as the outgrowth of an earlier school of Greek medicine—the priests of Asclepius. The Hippocratic physicians, however, opposed the Asclepians on several points and arose as a rival school.[4] Most importantly, the school of Hippocrates rejected the Asclepians' reliance on divine intervention to achieve a therapeutic result. Turning away from theological accounts of disease has been characterized by Ackernecht and others as Hippocrates' greatest contribution.

Just as important, Hippocrates and his followers were rivals of another school of medicine, located at the peninsula at Cnidus. Nuland tells us that the Cnidians "practiced a form of medicine that was in some ways more like our own than that of the physicians of Cos. The Cnidian focus was on the disease, while that of Hippocrates was on the patient. The

Cnidian physicians, like those of today, were reductionists" (Nuland 1989, 8–9).

Hippocrates, then, stood first of all for a philosophy of empirical naturalism, apart from superstition and myth. Secondly, he stood for holism, where illness was considered to be a derangement affecting the equilibrium of the patient considered as a unified human being, apart from tendencies to localize illness in isolated physical symptoms or causes. The tensions between Hippocratic philosophy and the philosophies of rival schools finds many analogies in the subsequent history of medicine.

In consonance with the Greek ethics of the day, the Hippocratic school conceived of kindness more as a good policy than as a feeling or an imperative to remain detached from egoistic concerns. The Hippocratic physician was concerned, among other things, with earning a good living; to this end he cultivated acts of kindliness and service to enhance his reputation and attract clientele. As Jonsen indicates, altruism did not appear as a distinct motive until the second century A.D., under the influence of Christianity (1990, 9).[5] The enduring presence of both the egoism of Hippocrates and the altruism of Judeo-Christianity is the first aspect of medicine's grand tradition to which I would like to call attention. Jonsen illustrates the current situation well in the following passage.

> Medicine is a skill so rare that it can be sold at a great price. Acquired with effort, it promises great rewards—not only of income but also of prestige, reputation, and gratitude. In this the modern physician inherits the Greek tradition. Nothing dishonest or shameful is involved, although, like any skill, it can be dishonestly and shamefully used. At the same time, medicine offers help desperately sought by persons hard pressed to purchase it. They, and society, expect that the help will be forthcoming. Outrage greets stories of the uninsured injured who are turned away from emergency rooms; incredulity is the reaction when rationing of medical care is mentioned. Stories of the doctor whose golf game or cocktail party delays attendance at the patient's bed arouse anger. For the modern physician inherits the tradition of monastic medicine: he or she is servant to "our lords, the sick." (1990, 10)

A second aspect of the tradition is its contrasting emphases on technological thoroughness and prudence. Following in the footsteps of illustrious pioneers such as Giovanni Morgagni, René Laennec, and Rudolph Virchow, Cabot devoted great effort to the education of physicians in the technical aspects of medical diagnostics and therapeutics. In Jonsen's words, he was interested in "the eradication of incompetence." As part of his general effort to improve diagnostic acumen, Cabot created an important feedback device—the clinicopathologic conference or CPC.[6] The CPC, now a cornerstone of medical education, met with frequent disapproval in Cabot's day, because it often exposed clinical incompetencies, which, in turn, threatened the self-esteem of physicians as well as public confidence in their abilities.[7] Cabot's reply to critics was partly that the virtues of honesty and humility are more important than the cultivation of a reputation—in this he reflected the previously discussed Judeo-Christian view—and partly that a reputation based on honesty and humility is eventually bound to eclipse the reputation built on concern for public image. But, most importantly, Cabot justified the CPC on the basis of the ethical priority of competence in diagnosis and therapeutics. Here Cabot echoed the thoughts of William Osler, who nearly two decades earlier had decried "a criminal laxity in medical education." In the same address, Osler stated:

> The aim of a (medical) school should be to have these (scientific) departments in the charge of men who have, first, *enthusiasm*, that deep love of a subject, that desire to teach and extend it without which all instruction becomes cold and lifeless; secondly, a *full personal knowledge of the branch taught*; not a second-hand information derived from books, but the living experience derived from experimental and practical work in the best laboratories. . . . Thirdly, men are required who have a *sense of obligation*, that feeling which impels a teacher to be also a contributor, and to add to the stores from which he so freely draws. And precisely here is the necessity to know the best that is taught in this branch, the world over. (1932, 29)

Osler goes on to encourage clinical teachers to accept the same sense of obligation.

That Osler should define the obligation of teachers in terms of technical and theoretical competence was characteristic of the progressive thinking of his time. The virtuous physician came, largely through the work of persons such as Osler and Cabot, to be viewed as one who had a command of the grandest and most up-to-date array of clinical skills and strategies. And, of course, the exhibition of virtue consisted in the employment of these skills. Competence, the comprehensive virtue, came to be associated with thoroughness. In the days of Osler and Cabot, self-imposed limits to the application of skills or technology were not a major question, and thoroughness was conceived essentially as a virtue without excess. Indeed, Osler commented in the above address that "the *Quality of Thoroughness*" was an element of such importance that he had thought of making it the sole subject of his address (1932, 36).

Lurking in the shadows of the emphasis on doing everything was the Greek ideal of moderation, exemplified in Aristotle's conception of virtue as the mean between extremes. In the context of medical care, this conception would dictate that skills not be employed in excess of reasonable limits. As medical technology became more potent and expensive, certain considerations of moderation came into conflict with the view of thoroughness as a virtue without excess. We will explore the genesis of this conflict in a moment. For now, it is enough to note that we have a development, exemplified by Cabot, in medicine's grand tradition that, coupled with a proliferation of technology, tends toward intensivism. One who venerates thoroughness—that is, the thoroughgoing employment of medical reasoning and technologies—is apt to act more aggressively, especially in difficult cases such as the care of chronically ill patients with serious complications, than one motivated by the ideal of moderation.

The medical student experiences the powerful influence of intensivism when he is assigned to the ICU, where he learns to create problem-centered progress notes that reconstruct a patient's illness into a series of clinical puzzles, to be solved by the appropriate employment of diagnostic testing and the arrangement and rearrangement of therapeutic modalities. Our student is apt, on occasion, to be repulsed by this arrangement, to question the prudence of reducing illness to a technical challenge. Such feelings are generated, at least in part, by an Aristotelian insight—the tendency toward moderation, which would subordinate the employment of clinical strategies to a higher vision of the well-being of the patient. This is not to say that Osler or Cabot were unconcerned with the well-being of patients. We shall later discover just how far such a characterization is from the truth. But, in their failure to foresee a future where moral limits to the growth or employment of technology are an issue, these thinkers helped to set in motion a way of thinking that has led to an important inconsistency in the modern form of medicine's grand tradition.

A third important aspect of medicine's tradition involves the development of ideals of respect for patient well-being and respect for patient autonomy. When I speak of respect for patient well-being, I refer not only to Judeo-Christian altruism, which views promotion of the well-being of patients as medicine's highest calling, but also to the Hippocratic notion that a physician's vocation is the application of measures to benefit the sick. What I wish to isolate is physicians' tendency—often derogatorily designated as "paternalism"—to see the benefit of the patient as a specific professional aim. This attitude contrasts with the view holding that the physician should be a tool of the patient's will. The two approaches conflict whenever the well-being of patients necessitates measures that are contrary (at least from the perspective of medicine) to their informed preferences. Although the Hippocratic oath contains a passage urging respect for privacy, today's concern with patient autonomy evolved largely under the influence of eighteenth-century liberalism, a school of thought with origins commonly traced to the philosophy of John Locke.

Locke and his descendants tended to view the individual—metaphysically, psychologically, morally, and epistemologically—as a self-contained being, endowed by nature with perfect freedom. In order to preserve their natural rights to life, liberty, and estate, Lockean individuals abrogate some of their freedom and form a commonwealth (Locke 1690, 66). The sole purpose of community, in Locke's view, is to guarantee the maximum freedom or autonomy of individuals, compatible with a lawful society where freedoms may be protected. That is, perfect freedom is abrogated only because it is insecure; the purpose of government is to ensure the maximum possible degree of secure freedom of individuals. It follows that the guiding moral ideal of liberalism is the freedom (or autonomy) of individuals. The traditional social role of the physician eventually became subject to modification as the implications of this view were recognized. Thus, in recent years the return to health has come to be viewed by some thinkers as the restoration of autonomy that was lost due to illness; and the restoration of autonomy is viewed by these thinkers as an imperative only if the patient autonomously wills it. By this account, physicians are not expected to be very concerned with the well-being of patients—that would be the patients' own responsibility. Instead, the physician is something of a hired hand, contractually obliged to help carry out the patient's will.

We have isolated three aspects of the medical tradition that represent loci of tension developed under the influence of differing schools of thought. The practical result of these tensions is the emergence of incompatible imperatives, leading to a dangerous fragmentation of medical ideals and a motivation crisis within the medical community. We turn now to a discussion of why these old inconsistencies have become such an acute problem in modern medicine.

THE EROSION OF THE ETHICS OF COMPETENCE

The ethics of competence is a system of moral ideals, principles, and practices. To a large degree, these may be summarized by the single injunction—"be competent." Two or three decades ago, Marcus Welby was a creditable champion of this system—a diagnostician of consummate skill, a devoted humanitarian, and an insightful ally of the sick, never failing to understand his patients' needs better than they did themselves. In family practice he was the descendent of Richard Cabot.

But the injunction to be competent has come to mean something different today from what it meant in the days of Richard Cabot. Let me represent the earlier and later meanings as S1 and S2, respectively:

S1: "Be competent": Adhere to a standard of practice that reflects thoroughgoing scientific rigor and humanitarian concern.

S2: "Be competent": Adhere to a standard of practice that reflects scrupulous attention to clinical and medicolegal consensus, i.e., practice according to the "standard of care."

Several factors preliminary to the metamorphosis from S1 to S2, all familiar, can be identified. First, there was the explosion of scientific knowledge. It is probably no exaggeration to claim that currently the corpus of medical knowledge undergoes more additions, deletions, and transformations in a single year than occurred in an entire century before Cabot began the practice of medicine. Several difficulties have attended this explosion: (1) It has become increasingly difficult to be a physician-scientist. That is, it is more difficult for physicians to care for patients and also to evaluate the medical literature with the sophistication expected of scientists. Richard Cabot may have known just about all there was to know about disease and its treatment in his day, but today no practicing physician can even approach effective command over the broad range of medical knowledge. (2) A result of the unwieldiness of medical knowledge and technologies is the proliferation of medical specialization, where medical knowledge is chopped up into manageable chunks and each chunk is assigned to a given specialty. Specialization compartmentalizes care. Compartmentalization diffuses responsibility and depersonalizes, from the standpoints of both the patient and the physician. (3) Of course, with the expansion of knowledge comes an expansion of technologies, and with the expansion of technologies comes increasing expense. Providing the best technologically possible care for all patients has become an untenable goal, based on the unbearable financial burden that would place on society. (4) Increasing invasiveness of medical care also comes as a result of the proliferation of technologies. Physicians and patients alike are resisting as barbarous the indignities and prolonged suffering that arise from the indiscriminate application of intensive care measures. (5) Finally, with the success of the "hard" sciences, the humanities have come to be viewed as "soft" and second rate.

A second important antecedent of the metamorphosis from S1 to S2 occurred in the field of the humanities—an increasing tendency toward relativism. Once again, the rise of ethical and cultural relativism is familiar. As the globe shrank and cultures intermingled, absolutisms of all forms came to be viewed with suspicion by enlightened scholars. Concern for the well-being or best interests of others came to be regarded as an act of presumptuousness. For the relativist, each of us sees the world entirely in the context of our own limited perspective. We are excluded from understanding the best interests of other persons, because their interests are a function of their several unique and inaccessible perspectives. Humanitarian efforts, in this view, are often acts of domination or exploitation— since to serve the "best interests" of others involves pigeonholing them into categories that generally accord with the worldview and the aspirations to power of so-called benefactors. One of the insights of the age of relativism is a widespread recognition that specific moral traditions, such as medicine's, are historically contingent. What unfortunately seems to have accompanied this insight is the conclusion that the moral views contained in such traditions are arbitrary, or at least not compelling.[8] Thus, medicine's ethics of competence began to lose its intellectual force. Student doctors, however deeply influenced by the tradition, came to find discourse or lectures about moral principles and obligations boring and irrelevant.

A third antecedent is the increasing tendency of the physician-patient relationship to come under the influence or jurisdiction of mediating parties. The personal closeness one found in Welbyan clinical encounters has been vitiated by the intrusion of legislatures, insurance agencies, attorneys, and hospital administrators; what is left is the medicolegal realm of the physician-patient relation.[9] Legislation such as COBRA[10], well intentioned but clumsy, ties the hands of physicians who wish to provide the best possible care expeditiously and diverts their attention from clinical concerns to legal concerns, burdening them with irrelevant paperwork.[11] Even apart from the interpretation of statutes, attorneys have found ways to control the practice of medicine—the emergence of a "national" legal standard of care being an important example (Young 1988–1989). Under the banner of cost containment, the federal and state governments have instituted a variety of clinical regulations and incentives, managed care organizations have proliferated clinical constraints, and insurance companies have devised their own methods of intruding into the process of clinical decision making (Morreim 1991, 23–40).

Each of the aforementioned trends stands behind the displacement of clinical emphasis from individual judgment to accordance with consensus. Corresponding to this displacement is the metamorphosis from S1 to S2. The emphasis on consensus is manifested by the proliferation of clinical guidelines and standards, often the end products of "consensus conferences." These conferences may be sponsored independently by various academic, legal, and specialty organizations, but occur ever more frequently under the auspices of organizations motivated primarily by the objective of containing burgeoning costs (Morreim 1991, 53–58). The modern physician often welcomes such developments. If thorough knowledge and sophisticated evaluation of the literature lies beyond the grasp of most clinicians, comfort comes in the availability of manageable general reviews and clinical protocols. In effect, most physicians have come to trust the judgment of recognized authorities in areas where physicians lack the time or ability to formulate basic clinical strategies through their own examination of the primary literature. Unfortunately, they have little control over the values guiding these standardizing inquiries.

Likewise, the modern accentuation of moral ambiguity has induced a reluctance to undertake moral calculations solitarily. Physicians who discuss ethical issues are more inclined to poll their colleagues than to develop sound philosophical arguments. Thus, at the 1993 ACEP Scientific Assembly the discussion of ethical dilemmas in emergency medicine consisted of about two hours of testimony—from physicians relating how they felt generally or how they reacted to one sticky situation or another. Evidently, the harangue was endured with the hope of attaining some sort of consensus on what is right but afforded no reasoned philosophical argument or even the introduction of a general philosophical viewpoint. Because a coherent stance on moral issues requires moral principles that cohere, generally on the basis of a logical relation to some basic philosophical insight(s), the attempt at solving moral dilemmas by the expression of more or less isolated feelings usually ends in no solution at all and with little in the way of a strategy for successful moral activity. With abysmal prospects in the field of ethics, medical personnel facing moral dilemmas have largely turned to attorneys for guidance, as if to say, "If we cannot agree on what is right, we shall at least adhere to what the courts prescribe." After all, legal opinions, though often devoid of philosophical sophistication, possess logical coherence and objectivity—qualities that have been lost from many nonjudicial discussions of moral dilemmas. The trend to replace ethics with law has become so pronounced that, at least in some circles, "medical ethics" has become a synonym for "legal medicine."

We have outlined, for now in summary fashion, some of the modern developments that have effected a metamorphosis in the ethics of competence. I have described this metamorphosis as an "erosion" because the new system, embodied in S2, is considerably less potent in dealing with the day-to-day challenges of medical practice than the old one. Though the old values that constitute medicine's grand tradition still manifest themselves in the self-understanding and emotions of modern physicians, they have been undermined by the accentuation of inconsistencies that have existed for centuries and by the recent popularity of relativism. Consequently, the elements of medicine's tradition exist in a kind of limbo. They lurk within the recesses of medicine's collective unconscious, affecting the medicolegal climate, or erupt from among physicians in paroxysmal sensations of a higher calling. But only infrequently are these elements explicitly referred to by practicing physicians, being out of fashion intellectually. They are displaced by preoccupation with clinical consensus.

As the battered tradition fades to the periphery, physicians are deprived of a stimulating ideal. Medicine, stripped of its nobility, seems at times to be nothing but one more means of earning a living. Emergency physicians especially are apt to view their work as a necessary evil, choosing their specialty because it allows them large blocks of free time in which to escape to a more rewarding life—perhaps parenting, recreational sports, an avocation, or a hobby. The profession as a whole seems to be suffering from what Habermas has called a "motivation crisis"—where the current ideals of the group have been undermined to the degree that they no longer command fervent devotion, where they lose their motivating power (Habermas 1975, 75). The metamorphosis from S1 to S2 is an erosion because it has weakened the tradition to the point of fracture. The elements of the old tradition no longer hold together. Even in the rare event where they are explicitly recognized, the moral foundations of medicine are apt to come across as a miscellaneous collection of mutually independent, ahistorical moral concerns, as in one of the current standard texts in bioethics, Beauchamp and Childress's *Principles of Biomedical Ethics*.[12] This fragmentation in ethics, as we have implied, results in a fragmentation in the self-image of physicians. Those physicians dedicated to practicing according to clinicolegal standards have divorced their professional life from their deepest moral beliefs. Where we once had the ideal of Marcus Welby, a humanitarian who unified his personal and professional lives through profound commitment to a moral ideal, we now have the perplexed physician of the nineties, bound by contradictory imperatives, wishing ultimately only to escape to the relative saneness of a fulfilling personal life.

But if the erosion of the ethics of competence is unfortunate, it is nevertheless clear that we cannot attempt to reclaim what has been lost in its old form. Marcus Welby never existed. And the ideal he embodied, though it emanated naturally, was never tenable. The grand tradition in medicine is a hybrid of various incompatible moral traditions, never quite rendered into a coherent whole. Tension within the tradition has been accentuated by modern developments. We must not forget that this tension will remain, no matter what we do to reclaim the past. In essence, the tradition has been eroded by external forces, but it has fractured due to antecedent structural weaknesses. If we wish to rebuild it—and it must be rebuilt if we are to escape the current malaise—then we must face the internal problems as well as the external threats. To this end I will introduce the ideas of Josiah Royce.

2

❖

Moral Ideals

■ In any moment of inactivity, great values are left unrealized through neglect. Whenever they are willed and enacted, they constitute a wealth which should not be underestimated. Our humanity is not so materialistic that it will always be expressed in idle talk. As I have come to know men, it has become clear to me that many more idealistic desires are present among them than become visible. Just as the waters of the visible stream are small in comparison to those which flow underground, so is also the discernible idealism among men in comparison with that which is unreleased or just barely expressed in their hearts.

—Albert Schweitzer

Josiah Royce begins *The Philosophy of Loyalty* with the observation that there is a modern trend toward the revision of traditions, reaching its climax in seemingly nihilistic theories such as Nietzsche's. Royce laments what in essence he describes as an identity crisis in modern culture, shaking the foundations of science, religion, and morality. Especially troublesome for Royce is the threat to the moral tradition:

But restlessness regarding the very foundations of morality—that seems to many of us especially discouraging. For that concerns both the seen and the unseen world, both the truths that justify the toil spent upon exact science, and the hopes for the love of which the religions of men have seemed dear. For what is science worth, and what is religion worth, if human life itself, for whose ennoblement science and religion have both labored, has no genuine moral standards by which one may measure its value? If, then, our moral standards themselves are questioned, the iron of doubt—so some of us feel—seems to enter our very hearts. (PL, 4)

The investigation that Royce offers in response to this problem is an investigation of the moral life of the individual. It is here that Royce hopes to find the foundations that will provide the basis of cultural stability as well as personal fulfillment. Thus, Royce begins—much as we did in the Introduction—as a sociologist, identifying the malaise of modern culture. But in PL he transforms into a psychologist, searching for answers to the general problem in the experience of individuals.

Royce sees moral standards as ideals by which we measure the worth of ourselves, our actions and our society. These standards arise out of a moral tradition. Thus, to revise a moral tradition is not merely to alter our appraisal of history, but also to readjust our self-image and our orientation to the future. When a community revises it traditions, it revises the ideals binding the members of the community to one another.

In the preceding chapter we summarized a series of changes affecting the tradition in medicine, and we indicated that further, more radical, changes are needed because: (1) in its current state the tradition is ineffective and (2) the tradition is inherently unstable due to internal inconsistencies. We turn now to the philosophy of Royce in the hope that an examination of how he approached the problem of revising traditions will help us identify the requisite changes. If Royce is correct, then much is at stake. If we undertake to revise the tradition in medicine, we are attempting to alter the ideals that unite health care providers and that give medicine whatever sense of community it now has.

Before we embark on this task, we should recognize at least two important alternatives to our program: (1) we could abandon the grand tradition in medicine and proceed with no ideals at all or (2) we could replace the grand tradition with another, entirely different set of ideals. Royce would eschew both of these alternatives, and it is worth our time to briefly consider why.

Regarding the first alternative, we have already come too far for abandonment to be possible. Although we have declared that certain aspects of the grand tradition are problematic, we have, in our development of these problems, demonstrated how the tradition in medicine is central to its practice. If we now go on to claim that we will abandon it and do without ideals, we deceive ourselves. Having no ideal becomes our only ideal. To make this move is to commit ourselves to the dubious position that, because we decide not to acknowledge them, our problems will go away. If we dispense with traditions, we dispense with the commitments that make medical research, medical training, and standards for medical care possible; the notion of quality improvement becomes incoherent. In short, we opt to strive for a condition of radical instability.

Regarding the second alternative, Royce would respond that our collective psyche is too profoundly influenced by the grand tradition in medicine to expect to radically escape its influence. With Peirce, Royce sees the attempt at starting from scratch—with a "blank slate," so to speak—as a symptom of intellectual naïveté, characteristic of the Enlightenment. For pragmatists such as Royce and Peirce, all meaningful theories unfold as interpretations of previous experiences, and, because the interpreted experiences are themselves interpretations, no stark experience or insight can be identified as something that exists apart from our historically conditioned modes of perception. Royce claims that even revolutions need continuity. He makes this point by observing, first, that the possibility for revolution is conditioned by the state of the institution against which rebellion will take place:

> Here the old has grown through successive apperceptions more and more complex. Each new epicycle added makes the mental work harder. At last the mind at a leap throws over the old for the new and simple apperception. *But if the gradual growth of the old from simplicity to complexity had not preceded, the revolution would have been impossible.* (LHE, 55–56)[1]

Next, he observes that revolutions are inherently conservative, seeking to reestablish the priority of selected, often ancient, elements of the tradition that is being overthrown. "Heretics," he notes, "are always trying to restore the ancient faith." To illustrate, he cites the French Revolution, conducted in the name of the "ancient liberties of the natural man," and the revolutionary ministry of Jesus, which sought to "fulfill the law and the prophets." He also cites Kepler:

> Kepler's revolutionary studies as to the planetary motions ended in apperceiving these as subject to the laws anciently demonstrated of the conic sections. Had this ancient doctrine not existed, he could not have used it and would not have discovered the planetary laws. (LHE, 60–61)

Let us dispense, then, with any notions of doing without a tradition, or of erasing medicine's moral history and starting afresh.

In this chapter we will discuss Royce's version of how individuals come to have moral ideals. Bearing in mind that Royce understands personal identity in terms of the commitment to moral ideals, this topic amounts to the story of how persons come to have personal identities.[2]

Royce on Imitation

Royce defines a human self as "a human life lived according to a plan" (PL, 79). To have a plan is, for Royce, to have an ideal; and it is through our pursuit of ideals that we achieve selfhood (WI II, 276). The process of idealization—that is, the process of becoming a person—begins at birth, and is, from the outset, a social process.

Royce's term for "plasticity in the presence of experience" is "docility" (OP, 35–38). Royce classifies intelligence as an advanced form of docility and considers a high degree of docility to be the hallmark—the differentia—of human organisms.[3] The "experience" to which human organisms are so adept at responding is not merely the result of interaction between the organism and its physical environment; it is, more importantly, a result of interaction between the organism and other organisms perceived as similar. In his discussion of docility, Royce begins with the observation that "man's response to his environment is not merely a reaction to things but is, and in fact predominantly is, a *reaction to persons*" (OP, 274). In the presence of persons, the human child itself learns to be a person.

It would be a mistake to look on the characteristic of docility as something predominantly passive. The docility of a human infant is manifested, in fact, through the distinct tendency of the infant to be active. Royce emphasizes that *acting* is itself a form of experience to which the docile organism adjusts (OP, 365–366). In fact, a human's responses to his or her own activities is as important in the formation of character as responses to other persons or to the broader environment. The energy or feistiness that characterizes the early years is an inherited characteristic, intimately related to social docility, which cuts across human cultures. Royce contends that "the foundation for our whole social consciousness seems to lie in certain instincts which characterize us as social beings, and which begin to assume considerable prominence toward the end of the first year of an infant's life" (OP, 275). He recognizes two major groups of such instincts: (1) those manifested in the phenomena of imitation; and (2) those manifested in the love of opposition (OP, 275–277). Acts of opposition tend to appear at a later stage of development than those of imitation (SGE, 185–186). Perhaps the choice of the term *instinct* is unfortunate, but the basic idea that the developing human person alternately manifests tendencies to imitation and to opposition is one that has been corroborated throughout the history of psychology and is reflected in the modern view, held by most personality theorists, that human personality expresses a developmental need for both identification and differentiation, the former manifested mainly in acts of imitation, the latter in acts of opposition.[4]

Through acts of imitation the human infant first comes to develop ideals of its own. Specifically, the infant's first self-conscious experiences of willing occur through the imitation of the wills of other persons, usually the parents.[5] The infant's perception of its own separateness or individuality does not occur apart from its perception of the individuality of others in its social milieu:

> As a fact, a man becomes self-conscious only in the most intimate connection with the growth of his social consciousness. These two forms of consciousness are not separable and opposed regions of a man's life; they are thoroughly interdependent. I am dependent on my fellows, not only physically, but to the very core of my conscious self-hood, not only for what, physically speaking, I am, but for what I take myself to be. (SGE, 201)

It may seem odd to speak of imitating the wills of other persons, and thus I will consider this process in a little more detail.

Will, in the wider sense, for Royce, is constituted of "the purposive side of our consciousness" (OP, 367) and permeates our entire conscious life. However, there is a narrower sense of "will" that is also important for Royce—"the attentive furthering of our interest in one act or desire against another" (OP, 368). This latter sense of will is an aspect of voluntary acts.

Royce does not think it possible to will what one has not yet experienced (OP, 369–370). Though this notion may seem implausible, we will see that Royce supports it powerfully. He thinks it is impossible to will to do something if one has not formed a working conception—through prior activities—of what one wants to do.[6] When the newborn cries, it does not do so because it specifically desires to be fed. The cry is, initially, a merely automatic expression of an inherited tendency—akin to a burp. However, after several cycles of hunger-crying-feeding, the infant undoubtedly comes to experience, in association with sensations of hunger, a desire or expectation for the feelings that come about in the act of feeding, and crying eventually becomes a willful expression of this desire. Thus, in even the most primitive act of will, the ideal is an object derived from past experience. The will to express ideas, to pursue goals, or to engage in higher order activities can evolve only under the tutelage of those who can impart an experience with these ideals. The young child wills to throw the football only after he has seen, and then imitated, his father or, perhaps, some player seen on television doing the same. His decision to become a Teenage Mutant Ninja Turtle is an act of will developing only after he has been exposed to other creatures who will the same and he has imitated their behavior in play. Further, insofar as he has not experienced the sensations of scaliness, of trudging around in a half-shell, or of engaging in genuine combat, the child's will to become a Teenage Mutant Ninja Turtle is actually only the will to engage in combat against imaginary bad-guys, in ridiculous attire, while using the terms "dude," "cowabunga," and "cowabunga dude" as often as possible.

As a corollary to the above consideration, Royce maintains that "before we can come to possess a will, we must first perform numerous and complex acts by virtue of the inherited tendencies of the brain" (OP, 371).

In essence, Royce argues that before we can possess a will, we must develop habits. The law of habit implies that "any conscious process which is of a type that has occurred before, tends to recur more readily" (OP, 198). Thus, repetition is an important antecedent to habituation and to willing. It is only through the combination of repetition and imitation that the child "gets acquainted with what he early finds to be the minds of other people" (SGE, 183).

One of the shortcomings of Royce's discussion in *Outlines of Psychology* is that it antedates his mature theory of interpretation. In WI, Royce divides cerebral processes into two categories: perception and conception. These processes are subspecies of what in OP he calls, respectively, sensitiveness and docility. To see how this dual theory of mental processes is inadequate, it will be instructive to examine how Royce deals in OP with the problem of spontaneity.

We have noted that Royce thinks it impossible to will what we have not already learned. This claim may seem obviously false. Specifically, it seems to be refuted whenever one wills to learn something new, to do something radically different from what one has done before or to act in any manner so as to realize a novel ideal. Royce recognizes this difficulty and addresses it in the following passage:

> One can indeed will an act which is sure to involve, in a given environment, absolutely novel consequences; but the act itself, so far as one wills it, is a familiar act. Thus a suicide can will an act which results in his own death, and so far he seems to be willing something which wholly transcends his past experience. But, as a fact, the act itself which he makes the direct object of his will (e.g. pointing a pistol and pulling the trigger, or swallowing a dose) is itself an act with which he is long since decidedly familiar. (OP, 370)

Royce may seem to be dividing the objectives of action into two groups: (1) the immediate action and (2) the consequences. He associates the first of these with the "direct object" of the will; the second seems to be only derivative of the directly willed action. Such a scheme does battle with our common perception that we frequently purpose the long-term effects of our actions more than the acts themselves. The medical student, for instance, has no experience of practicing medicine and, thus, by Royce's account, apparently wills not to practice medicine, but, for instance, to open his textbook and to study chapter 2 of Woodburne's *Essentials of Human Anatomy*. The fact remains that, for the medical student, the ideal of practicing medicine is what motivates his activity. Were that ideal absent, he would never pick up the textbook. Likewise, the suicidal person would never pick up the gun in the first place were it not for the desire to kill himself.

Royce's theory becomes more plausible, I believe, when we consider that even our long-term ideals are fashioned in terms drawn from our past experience. We cannot conceive of something wholly foreign, any more than the congenitally blind can conceive of redness. The blind may will to see colors; but I think Royce is correct to propose that what the blind actually will is the pleasure and excitement that often accompany novel experiences, and with these they are undoubtedly familiar. Likewise, the suicidal person does not will death; an individual in those straits wills the cessation of suffering. Royce's theory, so interpreted, seems to cohere with experience. On this account, original ideals are possible only in the sense of novel conglomerations of the familiar. However, novel experiences may result from such ideas; and thus the creative intellect is funded with an increasing supply of raw materials.[7]

Royce explains creativity, or "mental initiative," in terms of the "restless persistence" of human beings in arranging and rearranging ideas and in repeating acts not previously proved to be adaptive (OP, 318–319). In this discussion, aimed at addressing the problem of spontaneity, Royce verges on a theory of interpretation. The similarities with Peirce are striking. Both thinkers begin by acknowledging that thought is essentially adaptive; it is aimed at producing satisfactory actions in the face of various physical or psychological obstacles.[8] Both go on to cite restlessness as the parent of creativity (OP, 317–319; Peirce 1955, 10). And both acknowledge that the greatest advances—the most successful adaptations— are made when thinkers persevere in projects that seem initially to be non-adaptive (OP, 317–318; Peirce 1955, 48). Royce gives considerable time to this insight, carrying it far beyond the scientific plane of existence that occupied most of Peirce's attention. For instance, Royce illustrates how a child's persistence in non-adaptive games is an important aspect of its training (OP, 322,332). He stresses that this play is carried out not merely for the sake of pleasure but as the expression of an inherited drive: "as any close observer of childhood knows, children play, not merely because it pleases them, but *because they must play*" (OP, 322).

The whole context of this discussion presupposes interpretation as the predominant form of cognition. Though Royce has previously insisted on the purposeful nature of conceptions, and also acknowledged that our conceptions are funded by our past experience (WI I, 285), his emphasis on these aspects of cognition can be successfully carried off only within the context of a theory of interpretation. Specifically, only within the sign-cognitive or interpretive triadic paradigm of knowledge is the influence of social and environmental factors wholly admissible. Conception and perception are dyadic processes. Two elements are involved: the idea and its object. In such a dyadic relation, there is no room for the conception that the idea is affected by previous ideas or that it expresses a purpose rather than a simple relation of correspondence. Unfortunately— or, rather, fortunately—lived experience is too complex, too rich, to be portrayed through such a correspondence theory. Royce often speaks in WI as if humans were wholly occupied with questions of knowledge, as if truth were the unwavering goal of human endeavor. Expressing objectives—such as producing a work of art, walking in the woods, listening to music, or drinking a fine *Weissbier*—is at best awkward, if in terms of conformity to such an external, cognitive standard.

The theory of interpretation does more justice to these aims. The artist, for example, interprets an experience in a work of art. Three elements are involved: (1) the elements, drawn from experience, that stimulate the project; (2) the artist; and (3) the work of art. When we behold the work of art, another triadic process evolves, whose three elements are: (1) the work of art; (2) the appreciative observer (us); and (3) our impression of the work. It is no surprise, then, when Royce uses Homer and Beethoven to illustrate the process of interpretation (PC, 307). Even napping can be an interpretive process. It begins with a typical collection of sensory disturbances; we interpret these as sleepiness and head for the bedroom to take care of business. Sexual activities are frequently analogous.

OPPOSITION, CRISIS, AND THE BIRTH OF THE SELF

We have detailed the process by which human will, with its peculiar purposes or ideals, evolves from acts of imitation. We have also discussed the generation of novel ideals and explained the sense in which ideals come to express the creative stamp of individuals. It remains to be shown how individuals come to organize their ideals and how idealization is related to selfhood.

We earlier remarked that there were two characteristic higher forms of docility: imitation and opposition. We have dealt with imitation. But the child, as Royce suggests, can never come to regard itself as a unique personality through processes of imitation alone:

> But of course the child's relations to the varying non-Ego of consciousness do not remain merely imitative. When once he has other minds in his world, the function whose essence is the contrast between his conceptions of these minds and his view of his own response to them, can take as many forms as his natural instincts determine. He wants good things, and perhaps must feign affection or show politeness, or invent some other social device, to get what he wants. Here again is an activity depending upon and bringing to light, the contrast between his own intention, and the conceived or perceived personal traits and whims to which he conforms his little skill. He learns to converse, and gets a new form of the contrast between the sayings of others (which he interprets by listening), and his own ideas and meanings. He reaches the questioning age, and now he systematically peers into the minds of others as into an endlessly wealthy non-Ego, in whose presence he is by contrast self-conscious as an inquirer. Here, every time one has the essential element of contrast upon which all self-consciousness depends. Argument and quarreling later involve similar contrasts. (SGE, 185–186)

Royce considers social opposition to be, like imitation, instinctive, and he characterizes it as "love for contrasting one's self with one's fellows in behaviour, in opinion, or in power" (OP, 277). It is only through opposition (also a form of interpretation) that the child fully learns (1) that he or she is a unique individual, and (2) that uniqueness is manifested in terms of one's peculiar array of talents, abilities, roles, preferences, and aspirations. Thus, for Royce, it is through an interplay of the social processes of imitation and opposition that children come to have an identity of their own; and thus, "all the functions which constitute self-consciousness show themselves outwardly in social relations, that is, in dealings with other real or ideal personages, and are, in our own minds, profoundly related to and inseparable from our social consciousness" (OP, 279–280).

We have noted that opposition has a stronger influence later in the process of self-differentiation, frequently after personality structures gleaned from imitation are already well entrenched. In such cases, the intrusion of oppositional tendencies can be painful. A classic example is the adolescent identity crisis. Identity conflicts, major or minor, are an inevitable part of the development of a personal identity. They occur whenever conflict arises between consciously or subconsciously held ideals. An identity crisis occurs when identity conflicts come to dominate the psyche. As John Clendenning has remarked, Royce was a pioneer in the study of identity crisis (Clendenning 1985, 43). Royce saw the identity crisis as more than just a transient developmental problem, characteristic of adolescence. Identity problems were, for Royce, the impetus to human moral development. Clendenning cites Royce's letter to Stanley Hall: "Interest in the 'whole problem of reality,' involves, and means, an interest in solving the problem of who I am, of what I ideally ought to be, and of what my life means" (Clendenning 1985, 43; LJR, 368).

The inevitability of identity crises results, according to Royce, from the nature of idealization, with its alternating and contrasting emphases on independence and socialization, and from the central relation between personal identity and the good life. Royce, in his final years, identified what he called ethics' three leading ideas—autonomy, goodness, and duty (ECE II, 4). It is interesting to note how these ideas are at work during his "middle period"[9] in OP, RUL and PL. The notion of "goodness" appears in the natural inclination of persons to strive for a good life, manifested by a desire for a coherent and fruitful personal identity. Amidst the search for such a meaningful identity, the person struggles with the tension between individualism—exemplified in the idea of "autonomy"— and social responsiveness—related to (if not exemplified by) the idea of "duty."[10] This struggle is articulated by Royce in terms of paradox.

THE PARADOXICAL NATURE OF IDEALIZATION

As I have argued elsewhere (Trotter 1994), Royce views the evolution to selfhood as complicated by two apparent paradoxes. These paradoxes are generated by the tension between individualistic and social imperatives of personal development. Royce captures the individualistic imperative in what he calls the "principle of autonomy:"

> If you want to find out, then, what is right and what is good for you, bring your own will to self-consciousness. Your duty is what you yourself will do in so far as you clearly discover who you are, and what your place in the world is. (PL, 14)

This principle arises, at least in part, from psychological needs for self-differentiation. It seems that developing a will—that is, formulating one's ideals—is an essentially personal undertaking. A problem emerges, however, when one finds that the individual can never bring the will to consciousness through merely introspective processes:

> I can never find out what my own will is by merely brooding over my natural desires, or by following my momentary caprices. For by nature I am a sort of meeting place of countless streams of ancestral tendency. From moment to moment, if you consider me apart from my training, I am a collection of impulses. There is no one desire that is always present to me. Left to myself alone, I can never find out what my will is. . . . (PL, 14)

As we have illustrated at length in our discussion of imitation, the evolution of a will is through-and-through a social activity. We are everywhere dependent on others—our parents, our mentors, our friends, our heroes—to be our models. The social imperative becomes: If you want to find out what is right and good for you, if you want to develop your own personal set of ideals, you must consult your culture; you must situate yourself within an essentially social nexus. Obviously, the two imperatives—personal and social—lead to conflict. We feel that we must determine our moral principles autonomously, but by nature we do not have this capability. Royce concludes:

> Here, then, is the paradox. I, and only I, whenever I come to my own, can morally justify to myself my own plan of life. No outer authority can ever give me the true reason for my duty. Yet I, left

to myself, can never find a plan of life. I have no inborn ideal naturally present within myself. By nature I simply go on crying out
in a sort of chaotic self-will, according as the momentary play of
desire determines. (PL, 16)[11]

This is the paradox of self-realization. It is frequently manifested in
an oscillation between individualism and social concern. The adolescent,
for instance, yearns for autonomy and goes to great lengths to establish
his separateness from family members, as well as to eschew social roles,
such as "the good student" or "the star athlete," for example, that he feels
are thrust upon him. At the same time, he inevitably drifts into some new
social network, often manifesting his rebellion with an almost pathetic
conformity to the norms of a new group. Thus we see large groups of
teens, all dressed in the same "countercultural" fashions, all carrying cig-
arettes, all bantering in the same characteristic lingo. The adolescent may
develop a fierce devotion to his rebellious enclave, such as we see, in its
worst form, among the members of gangs.

What occurs, then, in the development of some youths, is (1) the ac-
quisition, through imitation and relatively nonconfrontational forms of
opposition, of temporarily stable social roles, (2) a heightening of oppositional tendencies, shown in rejection of these roles, and (3) the rapid acceptance of new roles. In this process, the differentiation to selfhood may
eventually result in a threat to the society that initially nurtured the self.
The German philosopher Karl Theo Humbach has isolated how Royce
expresses this tendency:

> The well-being of every individual human depends on his rela-
> tion to the community. Now when we inquire as to the way, ac-
> cording to Royce, in which one achieves this relation, we discover
> a paradox, upon which everything in question hangs: community
> is possible only in association with self-conscious being; self-con-
> sciousness, however, is a social-contrast effect and develops only
> where the individual treads inwardly and outwardly in opposi-
> tion to the community. . . . So we see that the individual who is
> awakened into self-consciousness is caught in a vicious circle; so-
> cial harmony is a condition for a meaningful life, social tension
> is a condition for self-consciousness and the knowledge of life's

meaning. The higher the cultural level, the more effective the education to self-consciousness, and the sharper the contrast to the community. The indispensable condition for every cultural development, the education to self-consciousness, thus contains the death-germ for every culture, namely the opposition of the individual to the cultural community. (1962, 129)

This is the second of the two aforementioned paradoxes—let us call it the paradox of social differentiation. It is essentially the flip side of the paradox of self-realization, viewed from the perspective of the community and its interests. Essentially, the problem is that opposition, necessary for differentiation and selfhood, naturally evolves into confrontation. Further, in cultures where differentiation is multifaceted and advanced, social confrontation becomes increasingly inevitable and intense, such that new forms of culture that threaten the old ones are constantly evolving. The result, viewed from the perspective of the social anthropologist, is a recurrent turning-in of culture on itself. As a culture advances, it creates its own countercurrents. The gentler countercurrents may be appropriated by a culture and have an enriching effect. But often, or eventually, the ripples of instability become waves of intellectual or physical revolt, and the culture is toppled by its own creations.

This account of the destructive effects of individuation is relevant to our topic. We are concerned with the precariousness of medicine's grand tradition, in its current form, and seek to remedy this precariousness by reconstructing the tradition. But, if all cultural achievements are destined to be eroded or overturned through the inevitable emergence of hostile individualism, our endeavor is misguided. The stability we seek may not be attainable. In fact, it may be that our attempts to forge a strong tradition will beget explosive rebellion. Royce notes, "soap bubbles burst, as we say, but never with explosive violence. Only strong boilers can do that. For they only can hold steam at high pressures. The strength of a revolution is measured by the amount of previous conservatism; and that is true in mind as in matter" (LHE, 57–58).

Somehow, if the project of reconstructing medicine's grand tradition is to succeed, the tension generated by these paradoxes must be lessened or resolved. On the one hand, society must develop a general moral ideal that is immune, as far as possible, from the kind of rigid, self-destructive conservatism that delivers moral life into the clutches of dogmatism. At the same time, it must offer enough guidance that moral life will not perish within the wilderness of arbitrary possibility, where moral sensibilities are stimulated first in one direction, then another, until our image of the good life is torn asunder by hopeless contradictions. Social influences should help children become unique individuals while retaining ties to society and its traditions, of fashioning and understanding their individual destinies in terms that include their neighbors. Parents and teachers should help them to integrate their solitude with the tumult of social life and to find peace and fulfillment in each. This challenge, for Royce, is the central problem for philosophy, and also for natural theology.

In *The Philosophy of Loyalty*, Royce identifies the assault on moral traditions as an important identity crisis. He is clear that it is not merely a national or collective identity crisis but one that leads to analogous crises of individuals. Our point about the moral tradition in medicine is analogous. For physicians and other professionals, comprehensive moral ideals are derived largely from moral traditions, and the functions of such traditions therefore parallel the functions of personal identity.[12]

The "double binds" experienced by our hypothetical ED physician in chapter 1 led to an identity conflict. That physician's self-image was positive—frugal and thorough, knowledgeable and compassionate. But our physician found that these identity components came into conflict, born not so much out of the physician's tendency to opposition as out of the desire to conform to professional standards (a sophisticated form of imitation). We suggested that the physician's problems stemmed from a faulty general moral ideal, that is, from the inherent instability and inconsistency of the current version of medicine's grand tradition. In view of our discussion of the paradox of social differentiation, it is no surprise that the polarity between egoism and altruism became a major factor contributing to the instability of this tradition. The task of revising the grand tradition seems clearly, then, to be an indispensable part of any remedy to the evils of medicine, from the perspectives of the medical community *and* the persons in it.

Likewise, Royce believes that the most fruitful general strategy for dealing with any identity crisis is to develop and appeal to a coherent, comprehensive, mediating moral ideal. The comprehensive ideal can serve as an authoritative identity component and, in this capacity, can serve as what Baumeister calls a "metacriterion" for sorting out and resolving conflicts between other identity components (1986, 26–27).

Ultimately Royce cites loyalty as the most satisfactory of such ideals. As we will see, the loyalist is one who defines himself in terms of his devotion to a cause. This devotion is an identity component, and it serves as a metacriterion of identity. For example, I may be an astronaut, loyally devoted—above all else—to the mission of exploring, charting, and annexing the surface of Mars and other remote areas of the solar system. If you ask me to tell you about myself, I will speak of my dedication to this aim. It is, Royce would say, my central or most important identity component. When I have to choose whether or not to get married, or to live in Houston or Albuquerque, I will make my decision in light of my commitment to this cause. As such, it is an important metacriterion. When Royce declares that "Your cause is just your own self writ large" (RPL I, 23), he has these considerations in mind.

But we must not look too far ahead. Loyalty is one among several prospective ideals of personal identity. To understand loyalty better, and why Royce finds it attractive, we will need to look at a few of these other ideals first.

Three Ideals of Personality

In RUL, Royce argued that the tension between autonomy and the social character of morals is not irresolvable:

> The two truths, (1) that nothing is right for me unless I will the end which makes this act right, while, on the other hand, (2) I never discover my own purposes without constantly consulting my social order—these two truths are not inconsistent. Their union, their interplay, determines the whole nature of ethical truth. (RUL, 273)

He attempts to illustrate how we respond to this tension by flirting with one ideal, then another, often drawing on diverse traditions. In a very general way, Royce summarizes four sorts of personality ideal, each containing metacriteria for choices concerning personal identity. His aim is to examine them and see how adequate they are with respect to (1) the resolution of the tension between individual and social aspects of morality and (2) the ability to sustain themselves through the seasons of moral and intellectual development. These ideals represent the "great types of personality which civilized man of very various nations and races have learned to emphasize" (RUL, 276).

The first ideal is that of the hero. The term *hero* is here understood in a somewhat specialized sense by Royce, as "a person who, in a given social order, is admirable or ideal by virtue of his great powers, of his great services to his community, and of the admirable and distinguished deeds by which he wins a kind of literal and worldly prominence" (RUL, 277).[13] One of the criteria for heroism, as here conceived, is social prominence. The hero is one whose deeds are known. He is an acknowledged, often celebrated, achiever. Royce frequently uses the term *stately self* to describe the hero, emphasizing the social rank that always characterizes this sort of personage. The hero is one who has been tutored within a stable tradition and who exemplifies the central values of this tradition. Every tradition is studded with tales of the exploits of its heroes, but certain cultures have seemed particularly to advance the importance of the hero. An example is the Greece of Homer, with its tales of Achilles and Odysseus. The Celts are another example. In the following passage, taken from an early Celtic saga, "The Cattle Raid of Cùailnge," the heroic obsession with fame is manifest:

> "A good day, then," said Cathub, "for he who takes arms today will be great and famous—and short-lived." "Wonderful news that," answered Cù Chulaind, "for, if I am famous, I will be happy even to live just one day." (Gantz 1981, 141)

Royce acknowledges that heroism of the sort just described is beyond the capabilities of most persons. Nevertheless, as an ideal, the hero is useful:

> Viewed as an ideal of personality, the conception of the hero has been repeatedly employed for ethical purposes. One sets before the young the story of heroic deeds or gives an account of the achievements of stately and dignified personalities, in order to define a purpose of living which is aroused in the mind as one

contemplates the fortunes and the powers of the great personality. It is true that one cannot say: "It is my duty to become a great or a distinguished or a stately personality;" for of course everyone knows that the hero's success, or the great man's dignity depends upon his inherited powers and upon his good fortunes as well as upon his moral activity. But one can indeed guide one's life by the example of the great, of the heroes, of the stately selves that any given civilization may delight to honor. Caesar or Alexander, or any other great historical character, may serve to define the purpose in life of one who does not hope himself to conquer either Gaul or Asia. One may, as they say, "burn" to be like the hero, as far as in him lies. (RUL, 277–278)

We have already portrayed one heroic personality—Marcus Welby. Welby is a man of consummate skill. His behavior and motives are everywhere those that are sanctioned by the community he serves, and his exploits are celebrated. What we have found with the Welbyan ideal is that it has not withstood changes that have affected the tradition he epitomizes. This failure is related, at least in part, to a flaw common to all similar heroic ideals.

If one fashions his moral ideal around the image of a hero, then worldly success, a prerequisite to heroism, becomes a criterion of moral worth. We have already recognized that fame or wealth cannot be a moral imperative, because they are generally not within the control of moral agents. Nevertheless, such matters of worldly success do, within the heroic framework, affect an agent's moral worth. The individual who burns to be like the hero is ultimately a success only insofar as he *is* like the hero. When heroism is used as a moral yardstick, individuals are found to be praiseworthy only insofar as they succeed in reaching their mark.

Among those of a given group whose members imitate, admire, or yearn to be like Michael Jordan, for instance, the one who achieves the most success on the court is likely to be held in the highest esteem—his opinions seem to matter more than the others; his friendship is more sought-after; he is more often asked to speak in public; he is more frequently praised. Through skill in basketball, this youth attains, at least in the eyes of those who pursue a similar ideal, a state of moral superiority. But, as any basketball coach will tell you, the more celebrated player is not always the player who has most faithfully devoted himself or herself to the game. Most individuals are incapable of ever playing in the NBA, even if they immerse themselves wholly in the attainment of this goal. Thus, some of the most herculean athletic efforts are rewarded with only modest success. The superiority of the sports superstar is no doubt predicated as much on talent as it is on moral attributes.

One of the problems with the heroic ideal, then, is that it understands one's moral destiny as something beyond one's control. Royce recognizes this difficulty in the moral ideals of both Job and Aristotle. An excerpt from the discussion of Job is instructive.

> Job's wonderful description of what used to be his own dignity in the days when God still showed him favor, is a wonderful example of a form of the ideal of the stately self. In the monologue here in question, Job conceives of his own moral perfection and righteousness in his former state of prosperity to have been intimately bound up, as things then stood, with his worldly status and with the esteem in which men held him. Princes then showed him reverence. Men were silent when he spoke. All praised him. And this was because both of his prosperity and of his righteousness. "Eyes was I to the blind, and feet was I to the lame." Power and beneficence were in those former times closely linked in Job's experience. His stateliness, the ideal beauty of his life, resulted from these. The pathos of Job's position when he uttered his lament is not only that he has lost his prosperity, but that his former ethical ideal has been shattered. (RUL, 281)

Physicians subscribing to the Welbyan vision of medicine have been a lot like Job. Whereas they have expected to live a life of beneficent service rewarded with wealth and worldly accolades, they have found it increasingly difficult to meet the expectations of their community. They have experienced a barrage of criticism, litigation, and hostile legislation, and, currently, many perceive that their incomes are soon to be substantially reduced. No wonder medical admissions committees have been so pessimistic about Welbyan candidates.

Marcus Welby, as a heroic ideal, is a failure because the modern physician who wishes to be like Welby is doomed to fail. This kind of ideal is especially apt to be damaged by social changes, because it belongs to an ethos which estimates the worth of the individual in accordance with a social standard. Marcus Welby is a hero not because he has pleased himself, not because he has lived according to a universal moral code, and not because he has strived toward the realization of some ultimate human aim. He is a hero because he fits into a sociocultural mold, because he conforms brilliantly to the fashion of his day.[14] When the fashions change, Welby is relegated to late-night.

The second great personality type is that of the self-denying self.[15] In the face of the failure of the heroic ideal, Royce notes that "the highly sensitive moral consciousness becomes aware that what I am is far from possessing that completeness and that peaceful self-control which I ought to possess." The formation of the second ideal, then, begins with an insight into the defectiveness of the human self:

> From this second point of view what I am is always so incomplete that it is rational to observe that by nature I am whatever I ought not to be. For if I were what I ought to be, my acts would conform to a single purpose. But by nature I neither know any single purpose of life, nor conform my acts even to such purposes as now seem to me to be the highest. The way of life, therefore, depends upon first learning a thoroughgoing self-denial. (RUL, 282)

What occurs, then, with the self-denying self is that it repudiates its own will; it reverses, insofar as such is possible, the previously reviewed process of developing a will. There is, paradoxically, an attempt to extinguish the will through an act of will. This extinguishment is accomplished by cultivating an attitude of detachment. The paradigm, for Royce, is the mystic. For Royce, the classic statement of the salient characteristics of the mystic is contained in the philosophy of Arthur Schopenhauer.

Unlike Kant, Schopenhauer believes he has access to the thing-in-itself. The thing-in-itself is will. But when Schopenhauer speaks of will as the thing-in-itself, he is not referring to the conscious will. The conscious will (what Schopenhauer calls a "phenomenon" of will) is merely a product of the will as thing-in-itself. Let us call the thing-in-itself the "metaphysical will" (this term is not Schopenhauer's). The metaphysical will is our essence insofar as we are equated with the thing-in-itself:[16]

> The will, as the thing-in-itself, constitutes the inner, true, and in-
> destructible nature of man; yet in itself it is without conscious-
> ness. For consciousness is conditioned by the intellect, and the
> intellect is a mere accident of our being, for it is a function of the
> brain. (Schopenhauer 1969, 2:201)

Time and space, for Schopenhauer, constitute the *principium indi-*
viduationis—the principle of individuation (Schopenhauer 1969, 1:112).
This principle is a manifestation of the metaphysical will, which itself is
outside time and space (and which, therefore, is not an individual). The
metaphysical will—the real—is not bound by law or necessity. Its manifestations are entirely capricious. Everything that exists is a result of its
caprice.

The conscious will, on the other hand, is generally schooled in the belief that it is an individual. It perceives itself as an agent *in* time and space
(though, in reality, it is an image of the metaphysical will that *generates*
time and space). The conscious will produces a "self," in the sense employed by Royce and Peirce, through a process of interpretation. Interpretation, of course, occurs only in space and time. The "self" of Royce
and Peirce was, for Schopenhauer, a mere accretion of the metaphysical
will. It is a production of the conscious will, laboring under the delusion
of its own individuality.

Such a self, according to Schopenhauer, is destined to suffer greatly.
The root of this suffering is desire. Desire springs capriciously from the
metaphysical will. Each desire is wholly arbitrary in relation to others,
which is to say, there is no central satisfaction that stands as a final cause
(nor a central desire that stands as the root) of all desire. But the self,
which constitutes itself teleologically by interpreting itself in terms of
goals and fulfillments, tends to view reality teleologically. Within such a
conceptual framework the self organizes and prioritizes desires. Particular desires come to be understood as derivatives of an intelligent, originative will. An attitude of optimism often results, founded on misconception. Such optimism breeds more pain, as the best-laid plans of each
self are squelched by twin perils: (1) internal inconsistency and (2) colli-
sion with the plans of other selves. The result is generally tragic.

Schopenhauer accordingly adopts an attitude of pessimism, reflected in the following passage:

> This world is the battle-ground of tormented and agonized beings who continue to exist only by each devouring the other. Therefore, every beast of prey in it is the living grave of thousands of others, and its self-maintenance is a chain of torturing deaths. Then in this world the capacity to feel pain increases with knowledge, and therefore reaches its highest degree in man, a degree that is the higher, the more intelligent the man. To this world the attempt has been made to adapt the system of *optimism*, and to demonstrate to us that it is the best of all possible worlds. The absurdity is glaring. . . . A teleologist then comes along and speaks to me in glowing terms about the wise arrangement by virtue of which care is taken that the planets do not run their heads against one another; that land and sea are not mixed up into pulp, but are held apart in a delightful way; also that everything is neither rigid in continual frost nor roasted with heat. . . . But this and everything like it are indeed mere *conditions sine quibus non*. If there is to be a world at all, if its planets are to exist at least as long as is needed for the ray of light from a remote fixed star to reach them, and are not, like Lessing's son, to depart again immediately after birth, then of course it could not be constructed so unskillfully that its very framework would threaten to collapse. But if we proceed to the *results* of the applauded work, if we consider the *players* who act on the stage so durably constructed, and then see how with sensibility pain makes its appearance, and increases in proportion as that sensibility develops into intelligence, and then how, keeping pace with this, desire and suffering come out ever more strongly, and increase, till at last human life affords no other material than that for tragedies and comedies, then whoever is not a hypocrite will hardly be disposed to break out into hallelujahs. (Schopenhauer 1969, 2:581)

Schopenhauer subsequently attempts to prove that the world is the worst of all possible worlds.

The impossibility of self-perfection follows rather straightforwardly, given the accuracy of Schopenhauer's account. Perfection is a state where nothing is lacking, where every aim has been reached. Since Schopenhauer holds that the satisfaction of one desire will always be followed by the occurrence of another desire, *ad infinitum*, he believes that the concept of a unifying *telos* is untenable. Any unifying final cause with enough content to motivate human action will be either unachievable or disappointing, since the achievement of any goal results in the satiety of the desire that instituted the goal. Satiety, by Schopenhauer's account, spawns more desire.

Given the dismal prognosis of the quest for self-realization, Schopenhauer opts for a contrary move—self-denial. We will not deal with the specifics of his program, except to indicate that it is predicated on the notion of detachment.[17] Schopenhauer's ideal moral beings are ones that view felt desires and activities as if from afar, as disinterested spectators. These beings reject morality based on moral principles and exhibit virtue founded on intuition (which is the source of true knowledge—knowledge of the thing-in-itself—for Schopenhauer). Virtuous activities are the direct embodiment of intuition, which operates only when a being is calm and detached. But insofar as it is detached, a being stands apart from the nexus of desires and plans that constitute selfhood. Virtue is not the virtue of a self but an expression of something far more primordial. Virtuous activity, in fact, is self-denial. Moral knowledge and virtue, then, go hand in hand with detachment and self-denial.

The problem with self-denying selves is that they are, despite aspirations to the contrary, creatures of this world. They must eat, sleep, work, and communicate. But if the goal of life is to escape selfhood, social activities, such as work, lose their significance. If people define themselves in terms of their professions, and other roles, then those who wish to extinguish selfhood must detach themselves from those roles. Life becomes, to say the least, something of a paradox or a lie. Religious mystics, especially those who hold that God's creation is good, must explain why they have been created, if the sole purpose of life is to return into the preconscious state of selflessness. Mystical religions tend to approach this problem in bizarre ways; most of them end up claiming that the world of persons, families, communities, pleasure, and suffering is not real. Buddha, for instance, begins his spiritual journey with the insight that life is primarily experienced as suffering. His disciples complete the project by concluding that suffering does not exist.

The self-denying self appears in medicine with almost the same regularity as the hero. Consider, for instance, Osler's advice to students of medicine:

> In the first place, acquire early the *Art of Detachment*, by which I mean the faculty of isolating yourselves from the pursuits and pleasures incident to youth. By nature man is the incarnation of idleness, which quality alone, amid the ruined remnants of Edenic characters, remains in all its primitive intensity. Occasionally we do find an individual who takes to toil as others to pleasure, but the majority of us have to wrestle hard with the original Adam, and find it no easy matter to scorn delights and live laborious days. . . . The discipline necessary to secure this art brings in its train habits of self-control and forms a valuable introduction to the sterner realities of life. (Osler 1932, 33)

The Judeo-Christian doctrine of human imperfection and the need for self-denial is prevalent in this passage. Osler's advice regarding the physician-patient relation also rings with strong overtones of self-denial—"we are here not to get all we can out of life for ourselves, but to try to make the lives of others happier" (Osler 1932, 368).

These attitudes persist strongly today. As we have discussed in chapter 1, they are often-conflicting parts of medicine's historical inheritance. The Judeo-Christian altruism of the grand tradition is antagonistic to the its Hippocratic egoism just because the self-denial of the former is contrary to the self-promotion of the latter.

But self-denial manifests itself in other ways besides altruism. It is also evident in the lives of medical professionals who seek to escape their professional personae. This development, at least on a large scale, is very recent. It may reflect a modern perception of flaws in the traditional character of medical practitioners analogous to the deficiencies in general human character that are expressed in the story of Adam. Just as self-denial came into prominence within Christianity because of the failure of the heroic ideal—expressed in characters such as Job—so I believe there is a modern form of professional self-denial resulting from the failure of the Welbyan hero. Professional self-denial, however, does not usually result in altruism. Instead, it generates alternative, non-professional, modes of self-development. Just as the failure of the heroic ideal led to an assertion of the worthlessness of the self, and, ultimately, the desire to exist outside the realm of social roles and structures, the failure of the Welbyan ideal has led to disillusionment, such as we expressed in chapter 1, with a resultant desire on the part of many physicians to exist as much as possible in a world outside the professional one.

This desire for extra-professional fulfillment is frequently embodied in the intense preoccupation with a hobby or avocation. I have known other physicians who defined themselves more as yachtsmen, martial artists, outdoorsmen, entrepreneurs, and even philosophers than as physicians. It is not unusual for such a physician to regard his work as mere routine, as an unavoidable process, necessary for existence. To quote Marx: "It [work] is not the satisfaction of a need, but only a *means* of satisfying other needs" (Marx 1963). Such physicians are obviously alienated from their work. But the source of this alienation differs from that of Marx's proletarian. The physician may, on occasion, be exploited. He is frequently coerced, by the intrusion of governing or corporate bodies, to work in ways that violate his will. He may be an intermediate man of the type described by Lachs, viewing himself as a mere intermediary in the process by which his patients carry out their will (Lachs 1981, 12). All of these considerations factor into the tendency to alienation or the denial of the professional self. Ultimately, though, Royce would hold that the denial of the professional self arises out of more fundamental flaws in the structure of this self, as an ideal. These flaws correspond to the ones we have identified in the hero.

Modern physicians, then, often seek detachment from their professional personae. In a limited way, they become self-denying selves—physicians who deny their physicianhood. The schism thus created is as troubling in this context as it was in the case of the mystic.

Physicians who discover the inadequacy of the Welbyan ideal—if they do not quit or construct an impenetrable emotional wall between themselves and their profession, or, possibly, after they flirt with these alternatives and find them also to be unsatisfactory—are quite likely to rebel. They will rebel against the conditions that led to the demise of Welby or rebel against the conditions that make it impossible to cloister themselves from their professional lives. This transition is, as we would expect, reflected in the fate of the self-denying self.

Royce explains the transition to rebellion in the following passage:

> The defeats that the stately self may receive from fortune, the hard lesson of spiritual faith that those who trust in heroes may have to learn, these, as we just saw, are especially a motive that have led in so frequent a definition of the righteous or rational purpose of the self in terms of self sacrifice. . . . But there is another lesson, that instead of this one, may be learned from the same experience. And this other lesson leads us to the third of the ideals of personality upon our list. One may say: "I am far from perfection; very well, then, at present my whole value lies in that individual and independent will by which I seek to get nearer to my own perfection. What I otherwise possess is indeed of no importance. But my own will, that at least nobody can take from me, and that is not mere possession; that is a creation, new every moment. My fortunes may be whatever they happen to be; the value of my personality lies in myself. I am dependent neither upon the gods nor upon nature, neither upon the good will of my fellows nor upon my worldly success, nor upon my stateliness, for what I really need. There is no good in life but what the rational will gives it. If one reads the lesson of life in this way one expresses one's ideal as that not of the self-abnegating self, but of the defiant self, the third one in our list of forms of personality. . . . Morality means self-expression. (RUL, 283–284)

To the student of philosophy, the connection between the defiant personality, so characterized, and the doctrines of stoicism should be apparent. Royce makes this connection explicit. However, there is another figure that Royce found to be the exemplary rebel of his day—Friedrich Nietzsche.[18]

Nietzsche unquestionably had a tendency to the asceticism of self-denying selves—an admiration, even a yearning, for self-denial. Yet he perceived the hypocrisy of self-destruction, that it was but a stage in a cycle of self-affirmation, a gathering of forces. To attach oneself too tenaciously to the ascetic ideal, was, for Nietzsche, to contradict the force that created the ascetic ideal; such was a failure characteristic of the weak. Nietzsche warns us that, if we are to be individuals, we must not "remain stuck" to our virtues or to our fatherland, as with the hero, or even to our detachment, as with the self-denying self. The avoidance of such attachments is, in fact, "the hardest test of independence" (1966, 52). To fail in this trial is to negate our own deepest impulse. Thus, he speaks to himself through the lips of Zarasthustra:

> Even in your folly and contempt, you despisers of the body, you serve your self. I say to you: your self itself wants to die and turns away from life. It is no longer capable of what it would do above all else: to create beyond itself. That is what it would do above all else, that is its fervent wish. (1954, 35)

Nietzsche was just as adamant in avoiding an attachment to the tastes that characterize the life of an aesthete. Always, for Nietzsche, there was a desire for creativity and originality. Though Nietzsche acknowledged the unseverable bond between the thinker and his historico-cultural situation, and in this sense preached a more sophisticated form of individualism than such earlier thinkers as Locke and Hume, it was always his goal to shake off, as much as possible, the shackles of history.[19]

Royce acknowledges much of value in the ideal of defiance. Of particular importance, for Royce, is the manner in which it expresses "one of the deepest insights of humanity, namely, the insight, that the self must always in the end be its own ethical director, and that the ideal cannot be defined merely in terms of fortune" (RUL, 285).

The problem with the defiant personality becomes manifest when one considers the fate of Royce's principle of autonomy. Royce refers to Kant in the context of his discussion of the rebel, and this is no mistake. It was Kant who brought the concept of an autonomous will to the forefront of moral philosophy. And Kant falls prey to the same fallacy as Nietzsche:

> Yet the ideal of a Titanic self-assertion hardly ever utters itself without showing that the whole value of this self-assertion can become real only in case there is a genuine life, having a social meaning, and a life in which the ideal gets a concrete expression. (RUL, 285)

Nietzsche, the individualist, must write. Kant must express his good will in social activity. Locke's notion of the pursuit of happiness is hollow if it is conceived merely as an activity of the individual in isolation. Just as Nietzsche's Zarasthustra ultimately views his life as one small chapter in the unfolding story of the *Übermensch*, Kant sees the culmination of his moral teaching in the development of a kingdom of ends. The individual, nurtured by the community, lives for naught if he cannot direct his energy back into the community. Even in the face of an eternal recurrence, the individual must situate himself within a nexus of personalities and recognize that however transitory his values, they are values only insofar as he expresses them to others, or at least to his future self. Why else would Nietzsche write or Zarasthustra speak?

The rebel can be a self, then, only if he tempers his defiance with the acknowledgment of some community of values—be it a community of expression, or some other relatively plastic social vehicle. Rebellion, as a fundamental moral outlook, is unintelligible apart from community. But at the same time, it is antagonistic to community and thus incompatible with selfhood.[20]

I do not believe that the rebel has ever been celebrated within medicine's grand tradition. One obvious reason is that the rebel, when he is widely accepted, becomes the standard. Because rebellion is rebellion against the standard, our rebel undergoes an inversion when recognized within a tradition. Certain popular caricatures of the rebellious physician—for example, Hawkeye Pierce or "the Fat Man" of Shem's *The House of God*—do not rebel against what they perceive to be the core values of the tradition. Instead, they lampoon the medical pharisees, the hypocrites who have lost sight of the central values because they are too concerned with their own personal prestige or wealth. Certainly, Hawkeye's prurient obsessions are presented as a contradiction to the Welbyan ideal; he is, no doubt, rebelling against an aspect of traditional medicine. But his behavior never compromises his fundamental devotion to patients, which is his centuries-old inheritance.

Camus's character, Rieux, in *The Plague*, may be the physician in literature who most closely approximates the rebel. Rieux is repetitively suspicious of high-flung ideals (1948, 126–127; 189; 197; 229–230; 271). He goes so far as to formulate his own striving in terms of a rebellion against creation (1948, 116; 196–197). Through fatigue, Rieux comes to reject his illusions about striving for a cure or helping the sick;

instead he stolidly does battle with the disease, viewed as a natural enemy and not as the affliction of any given patient (1948, 172). He experiences a social divorce:

> Had he been less tired, his senses more alert, that all-pervading odor of death might have made him sentimental. But when a man has had only four hours' sleep, he isn't sentimental. He sees things as they are; that is to say, he sees them in the garish light of justice—hideous, witless justice. And those other, the men and women under sentence to death, shared his bleak enlightenment. Before the plague he was welcomed as a savior. He was going to make them right with a couple of pills or an injection, and people took him by the arm on his way to the sickroom. Flattering, but dangerous. Now, on the contrary, he came accompanied by soldiers, and they had to hammer on the door with rifle-butts before the family would open it. (1948, 172–173)

Rieux has experienced the cataclysmic destruction of the heroic ideal. To a large extent, he wages his own personal battle against the plague, isolating himself as he releases others to their own peculiar obsessions (188). But, ultimately, even Rieux situates himself within the context of a shared endeavor. He tells the priest, whose doctrines he rejects: "We're working side by side for something that unites us—beyond blasphemy and prayers. And it's the only thing that matters" (197).[21] While he acknowledges to Rambert that he must pursue his own path, apart from aspirations to heroism, Rieux also comprehends a tangency between himself and Rambert—a common form of decency—which he describes as the only way to fight a plague. Rambert asks what he means by "common decency," and Rieux replies: "I don't know what it means for other people. But in my case I know that it consists in doing my job" (150). Rieux and Rambert will pursue separate paths; but they are united, at least, in being fellow pathfinders.

Royce concludes that each of the first three major ideals of personality has proved inadequate. The heroic personality defines its ideal almost wholly in terms of a social standard, and thus his moral life is inordinately susceptible to havoc wrought by the winds of social change. The self-denying self isolates itself so thoroughly from both its own individual tastes and its social milieu that it finds itself paralyzed in self-contradiction. The rebel, insofar as he effectively isolates himself from social influence, discovers that his individualistic machinations are meaningless cries in the dark, and he finds he must either return to social life or distill himself out of existence.

Royce proceeds from the failure of these three classical personality ideals to a discussion of the loyal personality. The transition comes in the final paragraph of the second Urbana lecture:

> So far then these three ideals give us a kind of circuit of one-sided expressions. Each ideal demands in a sense the other as a supplement in their completion. Is there any personal ideal which combines the motives of all these three? Is there any way of conceiving the self which is just at once to its natural dependence upon its social environment, to its search for an ideal perfection that lies beyond all fortune, and to its demand for independence of judgment, and for individual uniqueness of office? There is, I believe, such a personal ideal. It is the ideal that stands fourth on our list. It is the ideal of the loyal self. To its exposition, illustration, and defense, our next lecture shall be devoted. (RUL 285–286)

Let us proceed, then, to a discussion of loyalty.

3

❖

The Nature of Loyalty

■ And going a little farther, he fell on his face and prayed, "My
father, if it be possible, let this cup pass from me; nevertheless,
not as I will, but as thou wilt." (Matt. 26: 39)

No perfection, human or divine, stands apart from the hardship of
fidelity. This difficult fact insinuates itself from birth. If infants
were not endowed with aspirations to emulate the wills of their
parents, and the doggedness to carry out such tasks, young parents would
be well rested, but no infant would learn to walk or to speak. In athletics,
no championship is won outside the wake of pointed sacrifice and endurance, aimed at victory, conceived in terms of a tradition. No violinist
achieves virtuosity if not dedicated to mastering the predicating funda-
mentals. Community life—that is to say, *human* life in its complexity—
never varies on this point, though goals and commitments may often be
vague or ambiguous. Fidelity to moral ideals is nearly always afforded the
greatest esteem—not merely by those who agree on the worthiness of the
ideals, but often even by those who do not.

Likewise, no sin is more reviled than treachery. Benedict Arnold was
hated even by the English. Brutus and Cassius joined Judas Iscariot on the
brow of Lucifer, in the deepest ring of Dante's Hell.

Royce acknowledges the arduous character of moral fidelity but nevertheless holds that it is no mere burden on the road to goodness or excellence. It is the essence of the journey. It is the solution to the problem

of personal identity, and, ultimately, the mode of being with God. When, in devotion, we serve our neighbor or our community, both we and the others are transformed (PC 135). Through this transformation, a higher ideal is wrought, calling for the love and allegiance of each party. Our response to this call is our life of loyalty. Every loyal act fosters another transformation, and then another, until we establish infinite connectedness with the spiritual lives of other conscious beings. Through our fidelity, we become selves. Entirely devoid of loyalties, we would be as nothing. And when we betray our loyalties, we assault ourselves.

Such was the insight of Dante, I believe, as he fashioned the words of Fra Alberigo:

> as soon as any soul becomes a traitor,
>   as I was, then a demon takes its body
> away—and keeps that body in his power
> until its years have run their course completely.
>   The soul falls headlong, down into this cistern
> (Dante [Canto 33: 129–133], 307)

Deprived of its loyalties, the medieval soul could find no purchase in its worldly body; spiritual death preceded the body's demise. For Royceans, this story bears a timeless moral: We are all called to loyalty. Not to heed this call is to extinguish the most primordial human impulse; to betray it is to experience hell.[1]

Loyalty, then, is Royce's fourth and crowning moral ideal. In this chapter I will attempt to characterize Royce's concept of loyalty, and in the next we will examine Royce's reasons for favoring it over the others.

Loyalty Defined

Royce's preliminary definition of loyalty in the first chapter of PL is, "The willing and practical and thoroughgoing devotion of a person to a cause" (PL, 9).[2] Let us examine each of the elements of this definition.

A loyal person must have a cause or causes. The cause is something that the loyalist conceives as valuable for reasons that extend beyond its mere relation to self (PL, 10–11). It is something that exists, objectively, apart from one's own existence yet has a personal aspect:

Moreover, the cause to which a loyal man is devoted is never something wholly impersonal. It concerns other men. Loyalty is social. If one is a loyal servant of a cause, one has at least possible fellow servants. On the other hand, since a cause, in general, tends to unite the many fellow-servants in one service, it consequently seems to the loyal man to have a sort of impersonal or superpersonal quality about it. You can love an individual. But you can be loyal only to a tie that binds you and others into the same sort of unity, and loyal to individuals only through the tie. . . . Loyal lovers, for instance, are loyal not merely to one another as separate individuals, but to their love, to their union, which is something more than either of them, or even than both of them viewed as distinct individuals. (PL, 11)

The example of the lovers is particularly helpful if we are to understand what Royce means by "cause." Several aspects of his description of this relationship should be noted: (1) the lovers are loyal not merely to one another, but to a higher unity that comes about because of their relationship; (2) the higher unity is something with which each lover is personally involved, but its meaning and value are not exhausted by the individual characteristics of the lovers;[3] and (3) loyalty and love are related, but loyalty is not the love of an individual.

The cause is an ideal held by a social group. It is not the social group itself, except insofar as the group is defined in terms of the ideal—that is, insofar as the group is viewed as a community.[4] The distinction between loyalty as devotion to a specific organization and as devotion to the ideals of a community can be important. A wonderful illustration of this distinction, and its importance, occurs in a recent film.

In *A Few Good Men,* released in 1992 by Columbia Pictures, two soldiers are tried for murder. The facts of the case, which eventually come out during the trial, are essentially as follows: The soldiers are ordered by their lieutenant to visit the room of another soldier and to inflict a variety of minor tortures on him. They gag and restrain the victim, who was known to be a weakling, and, during the ordeal, notice that he starts to cough up blood. His tormentors desist when they comprehend his condition and call an ambulance, but he expires in the hospital.

Hazing of the type they inflicted was illegal but occurred with regularity at their station. When it was learned that the soldiers were acting according to orders, they were acquitted of murder. However, they were dishonorably discharged from the marines, for "conduct unbecoming a Marine."

The decision made by the jury in this case seems to be based on a distinction between the two types of loyalty I have mentioned above. In the first form of loyalty—what I will call "authoritarian loyalty"—the loyal individual is committed to fulfilling the directives of a person or group. We will call the person or group the "object" of authoritarian loyalty. The declarations, rules, and injunctions of the object are taken as authoritative, and it is the mission of the loyal individual to conform to them. The loyalty of the defendants was unwavering according to this standard.

In the second form of loyalty—what we will call "true loyalty"—the loyalist is expected to be devoted to the ideals of a community, a special kind of social group that is more than an organization defined by rules and procedures apart from overarching ideals. When one of the two marines asked the wiser of the two why they had been convicted of "conduct unbecoming," when, after all, they had only followed orders, he replied that they had a responsibility that transcended the responsibility to follow orders. It was the responsibility to look out for weaker individuals. The jury evidently thought that the Marines Corps was a community, committed to the ideal that the strong should protect the weak. In their estimation, the duty to be loyal to this ideal outweighed the duty to follow orders. They thought that true loyalty superseded authoritarian loyalty.[5]

In PC, the mature Royce defined loyalty as a certain species of love— the love of a community (PC, 119). This definition coheres with our notion of true loyalty because communities, in distinction to other types of social group, are defined by ideals. No set of laws, rules, hierarchies of command, or procedural principles can define a community. The ideals that define the community are the cause to which the loyalist is faithful, and the community is the "higher unity," described in the passage by Royce. We'll say more about the nature of communities shortly. But first we turn to the other terms used in Royce's preliminary definition of loyalty.

Loyalty, for Royce, is always an expression of will. Thus, Royce writes that loyalty is a *willing* devotion to a cause. In true loyalty, the cause is never something merely thrust upon an individual. It is chosen. Though a person's options are always limited by circumstances, the cause is never the person's only option. In order to devote oneself willingly to a cause, a person must recognize the cause as one among several alternatives and then choose this cause deliberately.

In the Pittsburgh Lectures, Royce says that the "permanent truth about individualism" consists precisely of the fact that the cause of the loyalist must be chosen personally (RPL I, 31). Royce here uses the term "individualism," or "ethical individualism," to denote the kind of thinking that arose from the ideal of the rebel. Ethical individualists, according to Royce, generally insist on one or both of two principles:

> (1) The principle that, about essentially important matters, the individual must in the end be guided, not by tradition, not by authority, but by his own independent judgment,—by his private intuitions, by his own inner voice, by his personal reason,—or perhaps simply by his mere determination to be free, to assert himself, and to win power; and (2) the principle that every individual has inalienable personal rights of his own, and that whatever duties he has must be in some sense made consistent with, and perhaps subordinated to these rights. These two, I say, are the essential principles of Individualism in morals. Briefly stated they are, (1) The principle of the freedom of private judgment; (2) The principle of the sanctity of private rights. (RPL I, 4–6)

In RPL Royce details the conflict between ethical individualism and traditional authoritarianism in terms similar to those he used in describing the tension between rebellion and heroism. He eschews ethical individualism for the same reason he rejects the ideal of the rebel, because he recognizes severe limitations in the degree to which individuals may be considered "independent." Nevertheless, Royce's qualms about independence do not result in a doctrine of determinism. He holds that each individual is unique and that we as individuals are free to determine which cause we will serve and how, uniquely, we will serve it.[6] When Royce says that our choice of a cause is free, he means that it is not causally determined in a strong sense (that is, in the sense that, given antecedent events, there is no other choice that could be made). When he says that it is not undertaken "independently," he has three things in mind. First, social conditioning (of the type discussed in chapter 2) is a precondition for choosing a moral ideal. Second, the choice of the ideal is affected by the social conditioning (that is, it is socially caused in the weak sense that the alternatives are limited by the social background). And third, the moral ideal itself must be a social ideal (which is to say, it must be the property of a community). None of these characteristics commits Royce to the view that the cause is not chosen freely.

Loyalty, for Royce, is a *practical* devotion. Never solely intellectual consent, it must be expressed in action. The cause must be served, not merely approved. With the pragmatists, Royce dismisses as meaningless any conviction or doctrine that does not manifest itself in the behavior of one who assents to it.

Finally, the loyalist's devotion to a cause is *thoroughgoing* in two senses. It is deeply ingrained and it is lasting. Again with the pragmatists, and with classical virtue ethicists such as Aristotle, Royce stresses that loyalty is a state of character. Loyal actions are the expressions of habit. The loyalist focuses so intently and so persistently on the sorts of behavior that the chosen cause requires that these behaviors become virtually automatic, as if they were hardwired into the loyalist's nervous system. They are elicited, almost without thought, when the appropriate situations arise.

True loyalty is expressed in the activities of a whole life. It is no mere posture or temporary disposition. One's devotion to cause is the hallmark of one's personality, unifying not only one's moral convictions but one's emotions and affiliations. It is the loyalist's ideal and deepest conviction. In defining the chosen cause, the loyalist defines his or her self. Royce maintains that the ties of loyalty are so binding that those who are truly loyal are willing to die for their cause (PL, 10).

Our basic sketch of loyalty can be filled in a little by looking at a loyal individual. My example is the German patriot Erwin Rommel.

ROMMEL'S NATURAL LOYALTY

On 16 July, 1944, two rather important events quietly took place in Europe, one on the continent and one in England. The first of these occurred at La Roche Guyon, a château near Bonnières, France, overlooking the Seine. It was here that Erwin Rommel completed the final draft of a letter to Hitler that he described as an ultimatum. The letter documented the dilapidated state of the German Army and the inevitability that Germany would yield the Western Front. In his own hand, Rommel added an audacious sentence: "It is necessary to draw the political conclusions from this situation."[7] Rommel made no secret about what he thought these conclusions were. He believed that Germany must make a hasty peace with the Western Allies and that surrender was in order. Though his opinion was branded "defeatist" by the Führer, Rommel had expressed it on several occasions. These declarations were anything but safe, especially in view of the failed attempt on Hitler's life—the so-called *Attentat* of July 20, perpetrated by Stauffenberg and others who were close to Rommel. In the wake of the *Attentat*, Hitler's paranoia increased, and his Gestapo went into an unprecedented frenzy, destroying scores of illustrious German patriots. More ominous than his pessimism about the prospects for holding the front, however, was Rommel's commitment to go behind Hitler's back, if necessary, in order to bring an end to the war. Rommel's letter was to be a final ultimatum. If Hitler did not make peace with the Allies, Rommel, backed by several associates, would take the necessary steps.

The second important event of July 16 occurred in England. Great Britain's "Special Air Service" learned of the whereabouts of Rommel's headquarters in La Roche Guyon, as well as his regular routes and routines. That day they received approval for an attempt to kill or kidnap Rommel. As David Fraser notes, "Opinion at staff level in the British 21st Army Group in Normandy had moved towards 'killing rather than capturing the gent in question'" (Fraser 1993, 512).

On July 17, Rommel's car was attacked by enemy aircraft and repeatedly strafed by gunfire. Rommel suffered a severe skull fracture, which debilitated him for the remainder of his life. He was permanently removed from the Western Front. We will never know what Rommel could have achieved had he not been attacked.

Rommel's biography is a case study in loyalty. In *Knight's Cross*, David Fraser writes:

Rommel's temperament, in private as well as professional matters, was essentially faithful. He valued loyalty almost beyond anything, and disliked the feckless, the changeable, the inconstant. Lucy was not only his wife . . . but for almost thirty years his utterly trusted companion and confidante, devoted, staunch and with a considerable sense of humour. He wrote to her daily—or as near daily as the exigencies of campaigning allowed. . . . Rommel had only limited interests outside his profession. He enjoyed sport, skiing, and other physical pursuits, and he always had an active and enquiring mind; but his inner absorption was in his soldiering and in his family. The latter provided a sure solace and background of loyalty and love, and it never failed him. His character was wholly dedicated and wholly faithful, wholly true. (19)

As a young officer, Rommel was tutored in the military philosophy of General Hans von Seeckt, who commanded the Rechswehr in the aftermath of World War I. General von Seeckt's policy was embraced wholeheartedly by Rommel: "Soldiers, of whatever rank, must play no part in politics and must have no vote at Parliamentary (or any other) elections. They must be well educated and of broad interests. But they must be loyal to the state and to the army itself, rather than to party or to any particular grouping of politicians" (Fraser 1993, 93). Rommel came, under the influence of Seeckt, to regard authoritarian loyalty as the highest moral ideal. Fraser, himself a senior British General, warns us of the dangers of this form of loyalty:

By the rigorous isolation of the army from the political process Seeckt encouraged in his officers and soldiers a certain political naivety. By law they were not to vote; but he also, as it were, ordered them to avert their eyes. He preached as the highest morality absolute loyalty to the state—the Fatherland—unadulterated by any partisan consideration, but he inadequately reflected that this dedication could make such loyalty vulnerable if the state itself ever conceded power to men themselves inherently immoral. He preached the absolute importance of obedience—the war had proved it: loyalty and obedience must not discriminate, must not follow private political inclination, even conviction. The state and the Oath must be binding and must be all. Yet loyalty and obedience can be betrayed. (94)

The political naïveté that was cultivated under this policy no doubt influenced some of Rommel's later actions. Rommel was, for instance, remarkably ignorant of the degree to which Hitler propounded and believed in a racial conspiracy theory (Fraser, 132). Rommel himself demonstrated egalitarian feelings about race.[8] It is ironic and tragic that a man such as Rommel could become an agent of someone like Hitler.

Late in World War II, Rommel largely overcame his naïveté. As he became wiser, his loyalty metamorphosed from its authoritarian beginnings. The Rommel who wrote the ultimatum to Hitler was a true loyalist. It is instructive to consider why.

From his earliest days of service, Rommel was devoted to Germany. For most of his life he believed that service to Germany consisted of living by a code of obedience. As we have indicated, such a belief is the defining characteristic of what we have called "authoritarian loyalty." But even as Rommel professed an ethic of adherence to procedure, he showed indications of a deeper respect for moral ideals transcending procedural principles. Of particular note was his lifelong and thoroughgoing consideration for the humanity and dignity of his enemies (Fraser 31; 44; 142; 180; 558). Also, Rommel's great esteem for the judgment of individuals, described by Fraser in the following passage, countervailed authoritarian tendencies:

> He was a fanatical believer in the importance of bold initiative by individuals. His own triumphs—and some setbacks—generally reflected this belief. Rommel believed that in battle success goes to the commander who seizes opportunity and exploits it; and that only he, rather than his superior, can perceive opportunity in time. His military philosophy, therefore, was one of encouraging, to the maximum, independence of judgment and action within an overall plan; and it was an independence which he exhibited from the first days of combat until the very end. For it he felt, then or later, not the smallest impulse to apologize. (43)

These sentiments, applied broadly to nonmilitary as well as military affairs, are echoed in Royce. Within the scope of devotion to a common ideal ("within an overall plan"), Royce believed that the maximum cultivation of individual initiative was a moral imperative. Royce's major criticism of Rommel would have been that he did not apply this rule broadly enough. He would have advised Rommel to take the initiative in broader strategic matters—which is to say, in the political and social arenas. Further, he would hold that acting on behalf of Germany's highest moral ideals is not enough, that Rommel must serve the ideals of humanity.

Eventually Rommel came to understand that the honor of Germany was not served by obedience to tyrants. Those who betrayed that honor, even those occupying the highest offices, were to be resisted and condemned. This belief is what animated his rebellion against Hitler. And it is this belief that Rommel expressed in the final hours of his life, as he confided in his son Manfred (Fraser, 528). In these culminating moments, Rommel, one of Germany's best-loved and most celebrated national icons, rejected the role of hero. He chose instead to be loyal.

On October 14, 1944, Rommel hosted two of Hitler's Generals at his estate. After a brief discussion, he went upstairs to talk to his wife. His first words were that he very shortly would be dead. He told her that he had been given a choice—suicide or an appearance before a people's court. Rommel instantly chose the former, guaranteeing that Lucy and Manfred would not suffer. Rommel then called on his son. He spoke briefly about Hitler's madness, the corruptness of the regime, and the duties of patriots. Manfred accompanied his father to a waiting car, occupied by his two visitors. Rommel wore his overcoat and cap, and was carrying his Field Marshal's service baton. Utterly calm, he bid his son farewell. Fifteen minutes later Lucy received a phone call from the reserve hospital. Rommel was dead. Of a heart attack, they said.

COMMUNITY AND INTERPRETATION: THE STRUCTURE OF LOYALTY

Loyalty is love of a community, which is to say, it is the willing and practical and thoroughgoing devotion of a person to the well-being of a community. What is a community? Royce writes:

> Now when many contemporary and distinct individual selves so interpret, each his own personal life, that each says of an individual past or of a determinate future event or deed: "That belongs to my life"; "That occurred, or will occur, to me," then

these many selves may be defined as hereby constituting, in a perfectly definite and objective, but also in a highly significant,
sense, a community. They may be said to constitute a community with reference to that particular past or future event, or
group of events, which each of them interprets as belonging to
his own personal past or to his own individual future. (PC, 248)

A community that arises out of mutual recollection of a past event is
called a community of memory. One that arises from mutual plans for the
future is called a community of expectation or hope. A healthy community will generally be a community of both memory and expectation.

If loyalty is devotion to the well-being of a community, then it is devotion to the tasks of vibrantly preserving the vital memories and achieving the hoped-for future that defines the community. These tasks are
achieved through a process of interpretation.

As I have explained elsewhere (Trotter 1994, 241–242), an interpretive process will contain three elements: (1) something interpreted, (2) an
interpreter, and (3) something towards which the interpreter (and, often,
the thing interpreted) aims. The term "interpretation" is used by Royce in
at least four distinct ways, as a designation for this type of process, to designate an individual instance of this process, as the function of the interpreter, and to designate element (3) above. In this study, I will refer to the
elements in this triadic process as the principal, the interpreter, and the
interpretant, respectively.[9] Each of the elements of an interpretive process
is a sign, where the term *sign* is understood in the Peircian sense as including not only physical icons, indices, and symbols but also the elements or moments—the Jamesian resting places—in the consciousness or
experience of an individual. The terminus of interpretation, element (3),
becomes itself a sign for future interpretations—that is, every interpretant
is, or potentially is, a principal.

Royce acknowledges Peirce as providing the model for his theory of
signs. Peirce's term "thought-sign" is illuminating. For Peirce, thoughts are
signs, in just the sense we have implied above. A brief illustration might
be helpful. Suppose I wake up at 4 A.M. to go to the bathroom, and, as I
traverse the dark hallway, I experience a searing sensation in my left foot.
This sensation, in the instant it occurs, is relatively unreflective: it occurs
abruptly and was unanticipated, and it is intense, so that it pushes other

aspects of thought beyond the periphery of consciousness. Let us designate this instant as T1 (Thought-Sign #1). In the very next instant, the searing sensation, which may already be decreasing in intensity, becomes the object of interpretation. That is, T1 becomes an object for interpretation in T2. I might exclaim, "Ouch," and in so doing I interpret T1 as an experience of pain. My exclamation at T2 (even if my "ouch" were nonverbal) is "aimed" at succeeding thoughts—its interpretants. I am saying that I have experienced pain. In this case, the message is relayed without deliberation, out of habit, but it is a message nonetheless. It establishes continuity between my present state and the states that precede and succeed it. Terms like *ouch* and concepts such as pain are reinforced because they are useful. The information they relay to future states of the self, and to other persons, will be utilized to make decisions.

The interpretation of T1 may be further refined. The T1-T2 complex can be taken as a sign in itself, and might be interpreted at T3 with the thought, "I've hurt my foot once again on one of Shane's toys." T3, of course, could factor into a whole string of eventual interpretations, for instance (Tx) my decision to bar Shane from playing Nintendo until he quits leaving his GI Joes lying in the hallway, (Ty) my wife's decision, when I return to bed, to hold off on asking me for a back rub, and (Tz) Shane's observation that the essence of virtue is to avoid being messy.

Of interest in the preceding example is the relation between interpretation and causality. Behaviorists would tell us that the "ouch" was caused by the pain—that it was a conditioned response. They are certainly right that it was conditioned. It was conditioned because its features are dependent on previous experience. They are also right that it was a response. They would say that it is a response to the spinothalamic stimulation initiated in Pacinian corpuscles in my foot. I agree, but add that it is also a response to previous thoughts about how to act in the presence of pain. If I had earlier decided that it was unmanly to express physical pain, this decision may have called forth—after a voluntary process of conditioning—a different response. Our "conditioned response," it seems, is an act by which we establish continuity with our past. In the moment it occurs, it may be experienced as essentially an involuntary spasm, but it also reflects decisions we have made earlier in life. T2 is not merely evoked. It is no mere result of physical events (or, at least, no behaviorist can prove that it is). It is also a product of my previous mental life, of my choices about who I want or ought to be. Further, as we will see, it is a means by which we call forth future acts.

The virtues are analogous to the so-called "conditioned responses." When Aristotle tells us that virtuous behavior proceeds from a firm and unchanging character, he is claiming that acting virtuously is, in important respects, similar to exclaiming, "Ouch," when one steps on a toy. The friendly man, for instance, does not stop and deliberate about what to do when he passes an acquaintance on the street. He automatically smiles and says, "Hello." But Aristotle recognizes that neither the "ouch" nor the "hello" is involuntary. Both actions reflect previous decisions and, probably, previous deliberation. They also send out messages. When I say, "Ouch," I tell the world that I am experiencing pain. When I smile, I tell my acquaintance I esteem her.

"Behavior modification," for Aristotle (and Royce), would not, or need not, be a passive affair. It may employ our powers of decision. Though we may need a teacher or a model to undertake a successful program of self-directed behavior modification, we contribute substantially ourselves. When we decide to take karate lessons, for example, we voluntarily undertake a process of behavior modification. If we are wise, we will visit several *dojos*, learning about the philosophy and policies of each, before we decide on our program. We deliberate about our objectives, and choose accordingly. During our training, we will practice certain techniques over and over, tens of thousands of times. We will rehearse the response to certain forms of attack so many times that, if we are ever put to the test, we will disarm our assailant without thought. One would not say, however, that our self-defense actions are involuntary. We have chosen our style of fighting. We have practiced certain techniques and neglected others. When it comes time to do battle, these decisions will have a profound influence on our behavior. By cultivating certain "conditioned responses," we project our will into the future.

Neither Royce nor Aristotle would claim that the expression of virtue is always this automatic.[10] Often we will be called upon to deliberate. My point is that, even in the most "thoughtless" behaviors—as in the exclamation of pain or a smile or the deflection of a blow—we act voluntarily. I have purposefully selected such automatic actions for illustrating the superiority of interpretation as a model of human thought. If it is superior to a simple cause-effect model for explaining behaviors such as these, it will certainly be superior for explaining more complex acts of cognition.

There are several other points I would like to make in reference to the example of stepping on a toy. First, not only thoughts but complexes of thoughts, some of which may be temporally disunited, may be signs. In our example, Tx is a decision that is reached only after taking stock of a lot of previous experiences and inferences. Thus, I might take several temporally discrete events as indicative of the attitude of my son, Shane, this past week and interpret them as a univocal sign that Shane ought to be punished.

Second, the thoughts of one person may become signs for another person. For instance, T3, the thought that "I've injured myself once again on one of Shane's toys," is expressed in my sanctions against Shane and in my demeanor when I return to bed. Both Shane and my wife may be able to decipher T3 from these clues. When they do, they are apt to interpret my thought, probably as part of a complex of signs, in the manner noted above. If I communicate T3 verbally, my words are interpreted as representing a thought of mine, and it is this thought, rather than my words, that is given weight in the future. Thus, we often forget the exact words someone speaks but nevertheless feel certain that we fully recollect the thought which that person wanted to communicate.[11]

Third, the interpretation of signs is an activity that is driven by human purposes; it is never a sterile analysis of the sign as it is in itself. In fact, as Peirce has argued, the qualitative aspect of the sign, the manner in which it exists for itself apart from a purposeful relation to other signs— in Peircian terminology, its Firstness—is unanalyzable. The immediate quality and intensity of the sensation I feel at T1 is, in itself, irrecoverable. No matter how vividly I describe it, I cannot convey or recover this feeling, any more than I can induce a burn on my hand by a vivid recollection of being burned. My interpretation of T1 is colored by several purposes that transcend it—my desire to avoid experiencing similar pain in the future, for instance, or my desire to teach Shane to be orderly and considerate.

Fourth, a stream of interpretations may be interrupted. In the previous example, a smooth and virtually effortless continuum of interpretations, beginning with my interpretation of certain sensations as the need to void, was interrupted when I stepped on the toy. At that instant the thought of going to the bathroom was wiped out of my consciousness.

With these lessons in mind, it may be easier for us to understand why Peirce (1955, 248–249) thinks that the human self is itself a sign. The rough-and-ready conception of the human self that most of us carry around probably coheres closely with the notion that the human self is constituted by the sum total of its life experiences. But, if each event in the inner life of an individual is a sign, and the aggregate of these signs is also a sign, then it follows that the person is a sign (both for herself and for others).

We have claimed that the love of a community is expressed through the activity of interpretation. This claim should be more comprehensible in light of the foregoing discussion. An individual becomes part of a community when coming to hold certain ideals (including both memories and expectations) in common with other people. Fidelity to these ideals is the instantiation of the individual's love for the community. In essence, the individual is a sign expressing the ideals of the community. Community life, then, is a relation between signs.[12]

For instance, suppose Lydia and Ian are dedicated to finding a cure for lung cancer. Both may have had relationships with those who suffer from the disease. Perhaps their memories of these relationships are mingled with convictions about helping others who suffer. And perhaps they are young students, talented in the sciences and faced with choices about a career. All these factors may combine to forge a commitment to lung-cancer research. At the time that they decide they will dedicate their lives to this aim, they reinterpret themselves—their mission, their reason for existence—in terms of an ideal that is itself, in part, an interpretation of their past life. When they recognize their partnership in this endeavor, their conception of their ideal and, likewise, their self-interpretations are transformed. The business of curing cancer is no longer a merely personal crusade; it is a tie that binds. Earlier, no doubt, Lydia and Ian experienced social motives and ties; both shared feelings of sadness or grief about the ravages of the disease. But in the shared resolve to discover a cure, a firmer bond is created. Lydia and Ian are related by no mere interest but by a firm mutual commitment to include: (1) a common identity component, (2) a common dedication to a cause, the realization of which they conceive to be more important than the fulfillment of any merely private and thus unshared aspirations, (3) a common vision of how the future ought to be (namely, free from the scourge of lung cancer), and (4) a helping orientation towards suffering humanity. Lydia's only aim is that the community realize its ideal. She will be just as content if Ian does the breakthrough studies as she would be if she does them. For herself, she only desires that she be faithful to her cause and that she play her role in a drama that exceeds her own life in its scope.

Lydia and Ian, if their attitudes are properly expressed in the preceding passage, are loyalists. They have formed a community, defined in terms of a common expectation or ideal, and love this community by interpreting their own lives in the manner indicated. Paramount in these acts of interpretation is the practical component. They express themselves by their actions on behalf of their ideal. These are acts of interpretation. Acts of self-expression are, in fact, always interpretations. They say to the world, and to oneself, "This is who I am."

Note that the fourth of the aforementioned characteristics of their mutual commitment renders the future professional lives of our cancer researchers into what is frequently referred to as a "calling"; their loyalties are their lifelong responses to the perception that their help is needed. We will soon explore how this humanitarian orientation is an aspect, for Royce, of all genuine loyalty. For now, it should be observed how comfortably the notion of a "calling" fits in with the sign-cognitive theory of idealization. When someone refers to her professional aspirations as the response to a personal calling, she situates her own life within an interpretive framework that features, as principal, that segment of the universe that issues the call.

The lives of Lydia and Ian are a continuous series of thought-signs. When they take on the mantle of their ideal, they unify these thought-signs by relating them to a higher purpose. No longer is either human individual defined in terms of a disjointed and tenuous continuum of thought—now she is a self; she has an identity; he is the expression of an ideal. But further, both individuals also unite their thoughts, through a common vision. It is in this act that a community is born or sustained. When the common vision is expressed in deeds, the community is served through acts of loyalty. We have claimed that loyalty is devotion to the well-being of a community, that it is devotion to the tasks of vibrantly preserving the vital memories and achieving the hoped-for future that defines the community. We now see how these tasks are achieved through a process of interpretation.

The Genuine Loyalty of Mahatma Gandhi

Recall the words of William Faulkner with which we began. We commented that Royce, like Faulkner, was committed to the elevation of humanity. The need to help, to be of genuine service, was one of the deepest motivating factors in Royce's life, and it is a key element in understanding the morally higher forms of loyalty. This need is expressed, perhaps nowhere better, than in Royce's letter to Elizabeth Randolph:

> Suppose that this world of people, all so needy, *needs my help.*
> Well then the question, Why must I live? begins to get its answer.
> . . . There is something I can do which no one else can do. That
> is: I can be friend of my friends, faithful to my own cause, servant of my own chosen task, worker among my needy brethren
> . . . but of course that *first* answer does not of itself tell you *what*
> it is which you are needed to do to help the other people. . . . It
> is just that purpose which I have tried, in my book, to define by
> the word "Loyalty." *The* help which my friends really most want
> of me, is help in living "in the unity of the spirit," as lovers and
> faithful friends, and patriots, and all those who together are devoted to . . . whatever *binds the souls of men in the common ties of*
> *the spirit.* . . . Whenever and however I can steadily and faithfully
> live in this way, I am really helping,—helping not only my own
> nearer friends, but, by my example and my indirect influence, I
> am helping everybody who is even remotely related to me or influenced by me, to give sense to his life. (LJR 548–549)

The movement from natural to genuine loyalty, to be outlined in this section, was fueled for Royce, by a deeply ingrained humanitarianism.[13] This strain of Royce's thought, exemplified in the above letter, cannot be neglected if we are to understand loyalty in its fullness.

Erwin Rommel eventually came to the conviction that his highest obligation was to preserve the virtue of Germany. To achieve this end, he needed to help other Germans to develop the same true spirit of loyalty that he possessed. Royce demands that the loyalist take this move one step further. We should, in his opinion, assist anyone we can in the cultivation of loyalty. Not just our countrymen, our coworkers, or our family—we are responsible, instead, to all humanity, insofar as we can effectively move them. For Royce, the highest obligation of the loyalist is the duty to promote the loyalty of fellow human beings. This duty is expressed in his imperative "be loyal to loyalty."

We have distinguished between authoritarian and true loyalty. Now we need to distinguish two types of true loyalty. Royce called the first "natural loyalty." Natural loyalty is the type of loyalty expressed by Rommel in his commitment to Germany. It is loyalty to the ideals of some naturally occurring community with limited membership. Natural loyalty is exclusive, cultivating and/or preserving a social division between its chosen followers and other natural communities. All of us have, or have had, our natural loyalties. These include the natural forms of loyalty to the family, to the professional group, and to the nation. The second type of true loyalty was dubbed "genuine loyalty" by Royce. This is loyalty to all humanity, where humanity is viewed as a (potential) community. There were shades of this form of loyalty in Rommel, exhibited in his behavior toward enemy prisoners, for instance. But, for Rommel, no ideal superseded the commitment to Germany. Loyalty to loyalty, on the other hand, consciously subordinates devotion to natural communities—that is, natural loyalties—to a higher devotion to humanity. When we make this move, our natural loyalties become genuine.

The community of all humanity is referred to by Royce as "the great community." "Loyalty to loyalty" can be alternatively expressed as "loyalty to the great community," or, as we now see, "genuine loyalty."

It would be a mistake to suppose that "authoritarian loyalty" was the only objectionable form of loyalty. In PL Royce claims that the best means of sorting out a bad cause (and, hence, of discerning a bad loyalty) is to determine if the cause is generally destructive to other causes. This criterion helps us to characterize two more forms of degenerate loyalty: (1) "militant loyalty," where the cause is served by directly assailing or destroying other loyalties (PL 27), and (2) "parasitic loyalty," such as we see in the mafia or in corporate raiders, where the cause is served by leaching upon the loyalties of others.[14]

I know of no finer modern exemplar of genuine loyalty than Mahatma Gandhi, and of no greater modern act of loyalty than his most famous political fast. To sharpen our notion of genuine loyalty, it will be worth our while to look at this event.

It is fitting that Gandhi's "epic fast" centered on the issue of India's untouchables. It would be difficult to conceive of an institution more at odds with the notion of a great community than that of India's ancient caste system and it untouchables. To call someone an untouchable is to exclude that person from any hope of membership in the community that you hold most sacred. According to the worldview of such a caste system, the notion of a great community, at least in Royce's sense, is incoherent.

But Gandhi was devoted to the great community. Gandhi prayed, above everything, for "the magnificent harmony of all human races" (Fischer 1954, 50). This ideal eclipsed even his commitment to India. He once said, "If India takes up the doctrine of the sword, she may gain momentary victory, but then India will cease to be the pride of my heart." Gandhi's commitments to nonviolence and to uniting Moslems and Hindus are legendary. Both derive from his commitment to the great community.[15] Nowhere, however, was Gandhi's passion for universal community manifested more dramatically than in his "epic fast" of 1932.

The fast was occasioned by a proposal put forth by an untouchable leader, Dr. Bhimrao Ramji Ambedkar, in the Second Round Table Conference in London in 1931. Ambedkar proposed to partition off a separate electorate for untouchables (referred to as "Depressed Classes" by the British). The proposal was accepted by the British, but protested by Gandhi in 1932. Gandhi reasoned that

> the mere fact of the Depressed Classes having double votes does not protect them or Hindu society from being disrupted. . . . I should not be against even overrepresentation of the Depressed Classes. What I am against is their statutory separation, even in a limited form, from the Hindu fold so long as they choose to belong to it. (Fischer, 116)

Gandhi had previously shown dissatisfaction with the caste system.[16] In 1928 he agreed to the marriage of his son outside his caste. He also accepted untouchables in his ashram. But on September 20, 1932, Gandhi made it into a matter of life and death. He promised to fast unremittingly until the untouchables were united politically with other Hindus.[17]

We will not go into detail about the events of the fast, nor about the political upheavals that attended it. Gandhi's fast lasted for six days, and he very nearly died. In the end, his requests were honored. The lot of the *"Harijan"* (meaning "children of God"—Gandhi's designation for the untouchables) was improved permanently, despite resistance he received from some of their leaders. He directed his fast not at the British, but at his fellow Hindus—urging them to follow his example and seek unity.

There are several aspects of Gandhi's fast that warrant mention. First, it was an act of genuine loyalty. Gandhi's loyalty to Hindu unity was an aspect of his loyalty to the unity of humanity. Second, it was, typically for Gandhi, an act of mediation. Through his efforts he sought to bring two struggling factions into harmony. Third, it was undertaken not so much for a political goal (Gandhi was willing to compromise on some, though not all, details) but for the ennoblement of the Hindu people. Fourth, he appealed to the better emotions of the combatants—their love—rather than threatening them. And fifth, it expresses the thoroughgoing nature of true loyalty—seen before in Rommel—in that Gandhi was unquestionably ready to die for his cause. Each of these aspects of Gandhi's fast distinguish it. Together, they make it the stuff of genuine loyalty on a legendary scale.

THE SPIRIT OF LOYALTY

Thus far our treatment of loyalty has centered mostly on Royce's early, provisional definition of loyalty from the first chapter of PL. This focus has been a function of the secular nature of our aim to amend medicine's tradition. Having sufficiently milked this provisional definition, I now alert the reader to some of its shortcomings.

First, it is too formulaic to suffice as a final definition of loyalty. Royce, in his later years, frequently expressed reservations about over-reliance on handy formulas, with its attendant intellectual hubris (RQP 141–160). Royce's fallibilism,[18] his insistence on the intimacy between cognition, affection and conation (Oppenheim 1993, 138), and his will to interpret, all reinforced his wariness about tidy abstractions. As we mentioned earlier, the later Royce came to express loyalty more frequently as the devotion to communities, rather than causes, just because the community was, for Royce, more concrete, more accessible, and more in touch with the dynamic nature of loyalty.

Second, the provisional definition of loyalty does not point sufficiently to the necessary connection between loyalty and communities of interpretation. This problem is closely related to the first. Once again, Royce was interested in underscoring the nature of loyalty as a living, growing relationship between individuals and communities. This organicity is less apparent in the conception of "devotion to a cause" than it is in "the love of a community."

Third, the characterization of loyalty as devotion to a cause is not responsive enough to the metaphysical elements of loyalty. This point has worked to our favor, since we are interested in keeping our discussion of metaphysics to an acceptable minimum. Nevertheless, not to acknowledge how Royce weaves the search for a functional personal identity with the process of ontologically constituting the self is to neglect a central aspect of his thought. The human self exists authentically only insofar as it embodies, through loyalty, the spirit of a living community. Only through genuine loyalty—where the human community is connected to an eternal, great community and, ultimately, nurtured by God, the spirit-interpreter—can the human person realize the true and complete selfhood which is, for Royce, the aim of life. In PL, Royce's final definition of loyalty is "the Will to Believe in something eternal, and to express that belief in the practical life of a human being" (PL 166). This definition is less productive than the earlier ones for the aims of this study. But we should remember that it tells us more about Royce.

Finally, the provisional definition of loyalty leans too heavily in the direction of natural loyalty, as opposed to the morally desirable expression of loyalty—that is, genuine loyalty. To express genuine loyalty in PL, Royce, not yet in possession of his mature conceptions of community and interpretation, had to speak of loyalty to loyalty—an abstraction that readers of this essay may already have found cumbersome. In later years, Royce was able to express genuine loyalty in more facile language: as devotion to the great community or love of the "Beloved Community" (which we will not discuss).[19] Royce went through over a dozen formulations of loyalty, altering them not only to fit his didactic objectives, but also to accommodate the increasingly fertile insights that characterized his final years. In this section we will examine a few of those insights. Hopefully, our excursion will be rewarded by a deeper understanding of loyalty, with fruits for our approach to the practice of medicine.

We begin deep within the hearth of Royce's life and thought, where vague stirrings of loyalty were wrought and honed by the flames of tribulation. From early childhood, Royce was intimate with the problem of evil. On a walk in the woods outside Grass Valley, California, the young Royce wandered among the remnants of a digging site and stumbled upon a miner's solitary grave—thus stimulating early thoughts about emptiness and death (Oppenheim 1993, 24). His early life was marked by all the hardships of frontier living, accented by a lack of physical robustness. One of young Josiah's acquaintances, Guy C. Earl, helps us bring the picture of Royce's early years into focus. Clendenning records that

> Earl emphasized the poverty and plainness of [Royce's] entire family. He remembered seeing them often at a Congregational church, ill clothed, homely, with strong family resemblances. He also remembered that his friend and one of Josie's classmates, Samuel Hall, once visited the Royces to inquire about the boy's prolonged absence from school. Finding the storefront after a good walk from the city's center, Hall was directed by Josie's mother to a woodshed in the backyard. In the shed you could see daylight through the cracks; there he found Josiah recovering from typhoid fever, lying in a straw bed on the dirt floor covered only by an old quilt. (1985, 34–35)

Later, enrolled in Lincoln Grammar School after a move to San Francisco, Royce—perceived not only as a quaint country boy, but as a preachy one as well—bore the cruel taunts of his classmates. Thus, before his teens, Royce had viewed or experienced evil in all of its general forms—as fear and emptiness, as physical suffering, and as moral depravity.

Not surprisingly, the problem of evil became something of a centerpiece in Royce's thought. No doubt, one of the aspects of pragmatism that attracted the young Royce was its acknowledgment that thought begins with a problem situation. In the realm of moral philosophy, the problem was the existence of evil. No pragmatist did more to address it.

In "The Problem of Job" (SGE 1–28), Royce considers the suffering of Job, arguing that it cannot be explained in terms of any of several pop-

ular responses to the problem of evil. The first of these—denying the teleological nature of the universe and thus explaining away evil in terms of
a neutral naturalism—had no pull for Royce and was dismissed without
serious discussion.[20] The second response was comprised of various attempts to mitigate the evil of human suffering by pointing to the fact that
painful experiences are instructive and help us to avoid future evils, including moral vice. This response was taken by Royce to be beside the
point, since the question still remained, why, in God's perfect creation,
did these potential future evils have to be an aspect of the universe? The
traditional argument about the relation between freedom and the potential for evil was a third response. Royce finds this avenue unsatisfactory,
since the evil that results from faulty human judgments is not the only
evil in the universe. It does not account for hurricanes or other "natural
disasters," nor for birth defects, or, to the point, for Job's wretchedness.
From here, the middle Royce offers the doctrine of absolute idealism as
the only viable solution:

> The answer to Job is: God is not in ultimate essence another
> being than yourself. He is the Absolute Being. You truly are one
> with God, part of his life. He is the very soul of your soul. And
> so, here is the first truth: When you suffer, *your sufferings are
> God's sufferings*, not his external work, not his external penalty,
> not the fruit of his neglect, but identically his own personal woe.
> In you God himself suffers, precisely as you do, and has all your
> concern in overcoming this grief.
>
> The true question then is: Why does God thus suffer? The
> sole possible, necessary, and sufficient answer is, Because without
> suffering, without ill, without woe, evil, tragedy, God's life could
> not be perfected. (SGE 14)

I will not go into the details of this solution. Of interest, however, is
Royce's conviction, expressed in this passage, that the path of virtue is one
of struggle, where human beings are together with God. Royce reports
that good, "as we mortals experience it," is something actively welcomed
or expected, which we "try to attain or keep, and regard with content,"
whereas evil is whatever we find repugnant and intolerable (SGE 18).
Good and evil are two poles of the only reality that one could describe as

moral. If there is something that we desire, then there is, of necessity, something shunned. To exist in a realm of no-desire, where everything is necessarily fulfilled in advance, is to exist in a nonmoral universe, where the notion of perfection could not arise. In the depths of our being, Royce tells us, our will is aligned with God's, and we struggle together—suffering, failing, regrouping—for the good.[21] No perfection is possible apart from this struggle. And total perfection is, from the perspective of humanity, always distant, on the horizon of infinitude.

The doctrines of SGE did not, alas, bring Royce to rest on the problem of evil. They were refined in PL, where Royce developed his notion of loyalty into the embodiment of the human response to God's eternal struggle. Later, in PC, Royce's concern over human imperfections blossomed into a doctrine of atonement that is one of the most powerful, if difficult, aspects of his moral philosophy. Though he develops this doctrine in the context of his discussion of Christian ideas, he views it as a necessary element of any mature ethics, writing that "The human aspect of the Christian idea of atonement is based upon such motives that, if there were no Christianity and no Christians in the world, the idea of atonement would have to be invented, before the higher levels of our moral existence could be fairly understood" (PC 165).

I will not endeavor in this study to defend Royce's theology. But his notion of atonement is worth our attention and should help us, in the long run, to carve a stronger version of medical morality. I leave to the reader's own resources to consider the ultimate problems of suffering, emptiness, death, and depravity and how they fit within the structure of the universe. It is certainly possible to construct a secular version of moral idealism that harbors a notion of atonement and affirms that, even though it be doomed, the quest for an eternal community is our only option. I suspect, with Royce, that such an enterprise can keep its momentum only by minimizing or looking askance at the horrible reality of evil in this world. From the vantage point of my own limited experience of evil—in the medical wards and elsewhere—I am not optimistic about the long-term prospects for a merely secular morality. But other thinkers of deep humanity, broad experience, and great insight—John Dewey, for example—would beg to differ on this subject. I will not engage them here.

The notion of atonement is not a comprehensive solution to the problem of evil. It applies, rather, to a species of this problem, namely to the moral frailty of human beings—including those who dwell within genuine communities. Let us call this the problem of depravity. For our purposes, this problem is constituted by the likelihood that any community, whether it be a small one, such as a family or local parish, or larger, such as a town, nation, or world community, is destined to be marred by betrayal. The human condition is such that this pitfall is inescapable. None of us is so strong that we are immune to temptation; and no community is so stalwart that it can successfully command the uncompromising loyalty of its members. Though we be fervent and devoted, our loyalty will never attain that purity which is our aim. Our lives and our communities will always be tainted by repeated failures.

In wavering from devotion, a loyalist, let us call him John, injures himself both in the narrow sense that John, as an individual, is compromised, and in the wider sense that his community, through which he identifies himself, has been irrecoverably harmed. In the wake of this treason, John, as loyalist, is apt to repent. But, Royce repeatedly tells us, no act of mere repentance on the part of the traitor, nor forgiveness on the part of the community, can undo the harm to the community nor relieve the loyalist from "the hell of the irrevocable" (PC 175). The deed will never be annulled. Nevertheless, Royce tells us, it can be in some measure reconciled. John's path to reconciliation is through the creative will of some other member or members of his community:

> . . . this triumph over treason can only be accomplished by the community, or on behalf of the community, through some steadfastly loyal servant who acts, so to speak, as the incarnation of the very spirit of the community itself. This faithful and suffering servant of the community may answer and confound treason by a work whose type I shall next venture to describe, in my own way, thus: First, this creative work shall include a deed, or various deeds, for which only just this treason furnishes the opportunity. Not treason in general, but just this individual treason shall give the occasion, and supply the condition of the creative deed which I am in ideal describing. . . . And hereupon the new deed, as I suppose, is so ingeniously devised, so concretely practical in the good which it accomplishes, that, when you look down upon the human world after the new creative deed has

been done in it, you say first, "This deed was made possible by that treason; and, secondly, *The world, as transformed by this creative deed, is better than it would have been had all else remained the same, but had that deed of treason not been done at all.*" That is, the new creative deed has made the new world better than it was before the blow of treason fell. (PC 180)

Royce notes that the Christian feeling is generally that Christ's work was so precious, and so gloriously transformative, that "the world as a whole was a nobler and richer and worthier creation than it would have been if Adam had not sinned" (PC 184–185). He also maintains that the problem of the traitor—and the general form of treating it—has "nothing to do with theological opinion on this topic. I insist that our problem is as familiar and empirical as is death or grief" (PC 179).

Perhaps Gandhi's epic fast was an act of atonement. The damage, in that case, was done by the Indians who sought to establish a form of political separatism, ostensibly on behalf of untouchables, that would be harmful to national unity. In view of the progress that ensued after the fast, as well as its inestimable inspirational value, it is quite likely that India—and the world—was, indeed, a better place because of the misdeed and Gandhi's subsequent atoning act.

I have argued elsewhere (1994, 263) that affirmative action, if we want to make it work, should not be viewed as an act of simple retributive justice. In this light it fails badly, and is, in fact, an inverted form of racism. Instead, it should be viewed as an act of atonement. Unfortunately, it does not seem likely that atonement is apt to be accomplished by a mandatory, government-backed program, and affirmative action seems to have contributed to a divisiveness of the sort that Gandhi foresaw in his own government's supposedly well-meaning legislation when he undertook his fast.

In health care, there seems to be a serious need for acts of atonement. We live in an unjust society, situated within an unjust world. How effectively could health care practitioners, should they be so inclined, help in the affair of atoning for society's manifold wrongs?[22] Further, as a group, physicians have benefited greatly from public trust—not always justly earned. Modern physicians can expect a thriving business. They are shielded from competition by restrictive medical school admissions, non-market-oriented fee determinants, and—in the case of certain lucrative specialties—a contrived limitation in the number of available residency positions, as well as by government-backed licensing and drug prescription regulations that restrict other, nonallopathic, forms of health care. In addition, they wield technology that has been developed largely on the strength of government grants. Nevertheless, the actions of the medical profession have, as a whole, been distressingly self-interested, betraying its professed loyalties to patients and to the larger community. In the latter chapters of this book we will look at ways we can right the medical profession and its moral tradition. But even if we are successful, the burden of prior failures will remain. Are there prospects for atoning these betrayals?

Medical practitioners would do well, I believe, to heed the famous example of Albert Schweitzer. His African work bears an uplifting, atoning spirit—expressed nicely in the following passage:

> By faith in the fundamental truth which is expressed in the concept of the "Fellowship of Those Who Bear the Mark of Pain," I established the hospital at Lambaréné. Above all, it affirms that whatever good we do for colonial peoples is not charity but atonement for the great suffering we have brought them from the first days that our ships found their ways to their lands. As we face them today, colonial problems cannot be solved by political measures alone. European and African must encounter one another in a new ethical spirit. Only then will understanding be possible. (Schweitzer 1965, 153)

The story of Joseph and his brothers is presented in detail in PC, as "the first instance of an extended account of an atoning process" in the Bible (PC, 202). That Royce should have selected this illustration is likely related to another trend in his later thought—an increasing emphasis on the family, both as a centrally important form of loyalty (WAR 36–38, 42–43, 56) and as a structural metaphor for related loyalties (WAR, 49, 71; ECE "Comments").[23]

In his Extension Course in Ethics, Royce models three general species of loyalty around three basic familial relationships—those between siblings, between spouses, and between parents and children. As with all loyalties, the loyalties exemplified by these familial relationships each manifest a synthesis of ethics' three leading ideas. However, for each type of relationship there is, in Royce's account, a most central leading idea. For the relation between siblings, the idea of autonomy is emphasized, since it is essential that each party be respectful of the other's need for relatively independent moral development. For spouses (as well as friends and lovers) the central idea is goodness. This relationship is that between relative equals, cultivating a happy, intimate life and sharing in the pursuit of common ideals. Finally, in the relationship between parents and children, Royce prescribes an emphasis on the idea of duty, where parents are responsible for protection and for nurturing the affections, virtues, autonomy, and wisdom of their children, while the children are expected to be appropriately obedient and respectful of family traditions (ECE "Comments," 11–32).

In our subsequent discussion of the health care community, these species of loyalty will come into play.

THE REVISION OF TRADITIONS

Gandhi's objective with the epic fast was to alter a tradition. The process by which traditions are revised is analogous to the process of revising loyalties—both types of revision occur when there is new information that indicates the current conception of an ideal, or how the ideal should be served, is inadequate. Traditions are the property of communities. When a tradition is revised, the loyalties of the members of that community undergo revisions—both the cause and the means of serving the cause are apt to change. Likewise, when the members of a community begin to experience changes in the way they conceive their ideals, or the methods by which their ideals ought to be served, and even if this change seems to occur apart from a metamorphosis in the tradition, it is inevitable that the tradition will eventually be affected. Currently, we find the medical community in a state where both loyalties and the tradition that supports them are undergoing profound changes.

Royce makes several recommendations about how and when to revise loyalties, and they correspond with recommendations about the revision of traditions. First, Royce advocates that we stand by a loyal decision once made, unless there is overwhelming evidence that it ought to be overturned (RPL II, 42–51; PL, 89). This recommendation is not so much about the revision as about the overthrow of loyalties, and, therefore, the strong note of conservatism it expresses probably ought to be tempered. The following rule would, I think, express Royce's opinion: Do not revise the ideal unless there is good evidence indicating a deficiency in it and good evidence that the proposed revision would be an improvement.[24] Second is the related recommendation that the ideal should not be altered more than the evidence requires.

A natural question arises. By what criteria do we judge an ideal to be deficient? Royce has three answers: (1) an ideal is deficient if it contains internal contradictions; (2) an ideal is deficient if it is shown that service to this ideal does not harmonize with the ideal of attaining a great community; and (3) an ideal is deficient if it has lost its motivating power.

These considerations lead to more recommendations about the revision of traditions. First, revisions ought always to be undertaken with rigorous attention to the matter of internal coherence. Second, the tradition ought always to be revised in the direction of service to the ideal of a great community. Third, revisions ought to be framed from a perspective that stimulates the activity of loyalists. We have, then, five rules about the revision of traditions:

(1) Do not undertake revision unless there are good reasons for questioning the ideal and good ideas about how to reform it.
(2) Do not alter the ideal more than necessary.
(3) When revising a tradition, attend to the matter of internal coherence.
(4) When revising a tradition, aim at service to the great community.
(5) When revising a tradition, try to fashion an ideal that will not merely harmonize but will also cultivate and sustain the loyalty of prospective members of the community.

The five recommendations brought forward in this section will come into play as we examine how medicine's grand tradition ought to be revised. But first, we need to provide structural support for our theory. We must explore why Royce considers his notion of loyalty to be compelling.

4

❖

The Need for Loyalty

I n the limited success of three moral ideals lie some important lessons. From the hero we have learned of the motivating power of social paragons. From the self-denying self we have learned that we are imperfect, that we must subordinate our baser tendencies and inclinations to higher ones, and that we must construct a moral ideal that will withstand the vicissitudes of fortune. From the rebel we have learned that we must be the guardians of our own moral destiny, that our moral ideals must be personal. For Royce, there is a moral ideal that combines the strengths of all of the previous three—loyalty. In this chapter we will see why Royce esteems loyalty so highly. We will discuss the "need" for loyalty from a dual frame of reference. In the first section we will consider loyalty as a psychological need—a hypothetical imperative—for the human individual who is confronted with the task of establishing a personal identity. Next, we will discuss how loyalty also becomes an ethical "need"—a categorical imperative.[1] This latter project will involve several steps. First, we will discuss the general manner in which Royce circumscribes the subject matter of morality, noting the fundamental importance he assigns to the attitudes of reasonableness and impartiality and how different grades of impartiality correspond to three levels of moral life. Next, we will discuss Royce's notion of moral insight. Through this insight, we will find, the moral agent is initiated into the genuinely moral life—the third of the aforementioned moral levels. Finally, we will discuss the ideal that arises within the context of such a genuinely moral life—Royce's concept of "loyalty to loyalty."

THE PSYCHOLOGICAL NEED FOR LOYALTY

In the second chapter we examined a central paradox. Beginning with the claim that establishing a personal identity (characterized as a stable, coherent set of habits and ideals) is a central aim of most human individuals, we discovered that, in Royce's words:

> I, and only I, whenever I come to my own, can morally justify to myself my own plan of life. No outer authority can ever give me the true reason for my duty. Yet I, left to myself, can never find a plan of life. I have no inborn ideal naturally present within myself. By nature I simply go on crying out in a sort of chaotic self-will, according as the momentary play of desire determines. (PL, 16)

This paradox—what we called "the paradox of self realization"—is the origin of a conflict between individualistic and social tendencies and is expressed in the flirtation with successive moral ideals.

We then examined some of the more prominent moral ideals that have appeared through history and that still present themselves as alternatives to the searching adolescent or adult. From a purely practical standpoint, where each ideal was examined as a hypothetical imperative designed to bring about a successful resolution to the problem of self-realization, the ideals all proved faulty. I suggested, with Royce, that the ideal of loyalty might provide a better solution. Then, in chapter 3, we developed the concept of loyalty as it is understood by Royce.

Now, we find ourselves on the verge of an answer to two related questions: (1) How does loyalty provide a solution to Royce's paradox of self-realization? and (2) Why is loyalty superior to the other moral ideals? The solutions to each of these questions, of course, will cover similar ground. Royce addresses (1) in PL, and (2) in RUL.

To overcome the paradox of self-realization is to still the raging battle between self-assertion and social conformity, without extinguishing either impulse:

> Neither within nor without, then, do I find what seems to me a settled authority,—a settled and harmonious plan of life,—

unless, indeed, one happy sort of union takes place between the inner and the outer, between my social world and myself, between my natural waywardness and the ways of my fellows. This happy union is the one that takes place whenever my mere social conformity, my docility as an imitative creature, turns into exactly that which, in these lectures, I shall call loyalty. (PL 19)

Royce illustrates how loyalty unifies the conflicts between self-will and social will with the example of the war spirit. He describes how an external crisis can transform the psychological state of one who is enmeshed in this inner conflict:

But now suppose that there appears in this man's life some one of the greater social passions, such as patriotism well exemplifies. Let his country be in danger. Let his elemental passion for conflict hereupon fuse with his brotherly love for his own countrymen into that fascinating and blood-thirsty form of humane but furious ecstacy, which is called the war-spirit. The mood in question may or may not be justified by the passing circumstances. For that I now care not. At its best the war-spirit is no very clear or rational state of anybody's mind. But one reason why men may love this spirit is that when it comes, it seems at once to define a plan of life,—a plan which solves the conflicts of self-will and conformity. This plan has two features: (1) it is through and through a social plan, obedient to the general will of one's country, submissive; (2) it is through and through an exaltation of the self, of the inner man, who now feels glorified through his sacrifice, dignified in his self-surrender, glad to be his country's servant and martyr. . . . (PL 20)

Before we expound on this example, I think several shortcomings ought to be pointed out in Royce's selection of the war spirit to illustrate the psychological value of loyalty. (1) As Royce observes, the traditional association between loyalty and the martial life has been, at least at times, "disastrous" (PL 7–8). (2) The war spirit is often a subspecies of what Royce later termed the "mob spirit," a degenerate form of loyalty where the spiritual progress of individuals is stymied.[2] (3) What we describe as the war spirit is often more of an emotional than a cognitive state; to the extent that the patriotic impulse derives from a sympathetic impulse, rather than empathetic insight, it is not, as we will later see, loyalty at all.

But let us suppose that the loyalty of our patriot is no mere emotional spasm. As he decides to serve his country, he begins to see the indignities and provocations that have been heaped upon his countrymen as crucial incidents in *his own* life. Through this perception he is transformed from a resident of his country into the member of a community, which is a community of memory insofar as each of his fellow patriots also takes these insults personally, and is a community of expectation insofar as each expects to set things right, through war if necessary. He is utterly enthralled by his cause, and it takes on the nature of a personal quest. Insofar as he serves the cause in his own unique way, he asserts his individuality while simultaneously securing his place in a grand social undertaking. He has reconciled the conflict between self-will and social will.

The patriotic loyalist exceeds the hero because he need not win personal renown—nor even survive the war—in order to count himself a success. Further, his cause will be just as valuable, just as satisfactory as a moral ideal, should the war be lost.

He exceeds the self-denying self by being a self. Instead of evading the challenge of self-realization, of giving in to the paradox, the loyalist overcomes it. The self-denying self abandons his project when he sees that it is difficult; the loyalist finds a way to cope and in so doing experiences fulfillment.

In distinction to the rebel, our loyalist is not isolated from the raw materials of inspiration and insight. In his ties with the community he enlists a cultural, spiritual, and cognitive resource that provides the needed structural support for individual striving. Unlike the rebel, the loyalist is not forced to deceive himself into believing that he can stand apart from these influences.

Loyalty, then, is good for the loyalist. An obvious question now arises. How, and in what sense, is loyalty morally good? It seems obvious that some loyalties—for instance, Lincoln's—are morally superior to others—for instance, Goebbels's. We have suggested that Royce differentiates between desirable and undesirable forms of loyalty by appealing to the notion of a great community. What is the justification for this notion? These are the questions I will seek to answer in the following sections.

THE MORAL LIFE: LOYALTY AS AN ETHICAL NEED

Not all behavior is moral. Nonmoral or premoral behavior is, for Royce and others in the pragmatist tradition, impulse-driven behavior. This sort of behavior is generally attributed to animals. When an impulse comes, it is acted upon, unless there is another, stronger impulse, in which case the latter is acted upon.

The realm of moral behavior is demarcated, for Royce as for Dewey, by the operation of intelligence. That is to say, moral behavior is reflective behavior. When one becomes capable of making a plan and following it, one is capable of moral behavior. Royce seems to recognize three very general and vaguely demarcated levels of moral life: (1) where one's plans are conceived individualistically, (2) where one's plans are conceived in terms of the realization of the aims of a favored group, and (3) where one's plans are organized around a conception of the good of all humanity.

Note that the aforementioned levels are differentiated on the basis of diverging general modes of viewing the moral landscape. At the first level, human affairs are viewed through the lens of self-interest. At the second level, the interests of a favored group hold sway. Finally, at the third level, one's vision is unclouded and expansive; localized interests are viewed in the context of an ideal of organically unified human activity. According to Royce, then, human affairs can be viewed from at least three perspectives. Let us refer to these three perspectives as moral vistas. The three moral vistas correspond to the three levels of moral life. One's moral life—that nexus of activity including one's actions and intentions—is, in part, a function of one's perspective.

By the term "perspective," I refer to one's unique frame of reference. One's perspective includes not only the general mode in which one views the world—characterized in terms of one of the three moral vistas—but also more specific personal characteristics. One's perspective, broadly viewed, is a product of one's entire life experience. Perhaps John Dewey was the most diligent of pragmatist philosophers in insisting that each of the aspects of mental life—thoughts, perceptions, plans, and feelings—

are influenced by our past. In his terms, "experience is funded." Royce would agree. A perspective, for Royce as for Dewey, is a store of dispositions or habits—dispositions to think in certain ways, to see or experience things in certain ways, to respond to difficulties in certain ways—that have accumulated through time. A few of these dispositions may be largely inherited or instinctive, most are acquired.

Just as one's life plan, in whatever form it materializes, is a crucial constituent of one's perspective, one's perspective affects how one develops a life plan. Royce's three moral vistas are, indeed, three general ways of viewing the life plan. An analogy to MacIntyre's notion of narratives is apparent at this point. The life plan, for Royce, is a conceptual framework through which one constructs an account of one's life—a moral narrative. The three levels of moral life correspond to three different general types of moral narrative.

The life plan, using Baumeister's terminology, provides both continuity and differentiation. It is a central, almost comprehensive, identity component. In addition, it is a metacriterion of other identity components, as well as of itself. As an illustration, consider a young woman who plans to devote her professional life to the development of a cure for multiple sclerosis. This plan will no doubt be a metacriterion for her choice between two possible university positions—it will cause her to ask which university is more committed to research in MS. Once she decides, her life plan will be more determinant—it will be to develop a cure for MS in her capacity as a researcher at the chosen university. The life plan, in this instance, has served as a metacriterion for itself. In just this sense, the life plan is a self-regulating aspect of personal identity.

There are two important prerequisites to the formation of a plan. The first is that one develop a complex of attitudes and abilities that Royce designates by the term *reasonableness*. These include the analytic ability to view various impulses and desires abstractly and objectively, as distinct facts or objective values, along with the synthetic ability of recognizing their connectedness in a space-time continuum. Also included is the ability to compare them and reason about them. The second prerequisite is that one develop an attitude of *impartiality*, defined as the recognition that all desires, impulses, and ideals are values that are, prima facie, worthy of respect.

At the first level of moral life, where one's plans are conceived from an individualistic frame of reference—an outlook Royce often refers to as "selfishness"—the virtuous life is a life of prudence. This individual's plans are designed with his own well-being the uppermost concern. He must be self-aware to the degree that he can evaluate, compare, and prioritize his own desires or interests and develop strategies for self-fulfillment. To accomplish this task, he must learn to be objective about the relative merits of his own various desires. He must learn to avoid those indulgences that will interfere with the attainment of higher-level ideals, and he must take the ideals of other persons into account only insofar as it is necessary to achieve his own ends. The Epicureans would be, for Royce, an example of a philosophical school that understood morality from this frame of reference (RAP, 37).

The second level of moral life, where our individual is concerned with the realization of the aims of a favored group, is the realm of loyalty as it is traditionally conceived, the realm of natural loyalty. Here, our individual subordinates personal desires to the interests of the group.[3] In this sense, the moral agent may no longer be regarded as selfish. Yet, in another sense, he may still be profoundly selfish. If he is an ardent nationalist, who pledges fidelity to an ethnic or cultural group, and is willing to pursue the purposes of this group even when they confound the legitimate aims of a much wider segment of humanity, he is selfish in that it is *his* group with which he is concerned. In place of an individualism of persons, such thinkers conceive the world in terms of an individualism of groups. The interests of other groups are taken into account only insofar as this is necessary to promote the welfare of the favored group. The analogy with the first level is obvious. A thinker at this level must grant an impartial prima facie legitimacy to his own personal interests and to those of his group. Though he has extended his scope of moral concern—he will take more into account when he deliberates about what is right or what is best than the narrowly selfish person—he nevertheless is concerned only with a small section of humanity.

Genuine loyalty occurs at the third level of moral life. Here, our individual as moral agent subordinates his loyalty to various communities to his loyalty to humanity. The values or ideals of all persons are respected. The competition between selves and between groups is mediated by the view that whatever furthers the interests of humanity as a whole, to whatever degree, is superior in just that degree over that which does not. Every desire, every impulse, as well as all the ideals that emanate from human activity, are considered with only one conscious "bias"—that humanity should be served.

There are several important points that should be brought out regarding the notion of impartiality here employed. First, to view competing values impartially does not require that we view them as moral equals. When we grant prima facie legitimacy to an ideal, we acknowledge that we will not discredit it because of its source. In this act, we assure that the ideal will be examined on its own merit and considered valid until it is shown otherwise through the application of standards that apply equally to all other values. Thus, to say that Hitler's ideal of mass murder will be respected equally alongside Schiller's ideal of universal brotherhood is not to say that we will condone mass murder, only that if we reject mass murder while advocating universal brotherhood, it will be because the former does not adequately measure up to the objective standards met by the latter. It is to say that we will not write off Hitler's ideals out of an arbitrary (nonmoral) bias against Hitler or his culture.

Second, Royce's notion of impartiality is united to his notion of objectivity. In general, when we say of a judgment that it is "objective," we imply that it is free of bias. Royce would hold that bias, in a moral judgment, would consist of an appeal to some standard or ideal that is unrelated to the ideals of a universal human community. Ultimately, objective standards are standards that belong to the great community. They are the habits of thought that would emerge out of an infinite process of interpretation. Royce, with Peirce, views the ideal moral community as a fully harmonious community of interpretation. Inner experience would be radically different in such a community. Every object—including every moral agent—would be fully interpreted, and thus our experience of objects would no longer be of the nature of an encounter. Every being would be transparent to him- or herself and others. In fact, the selfhood of moral agents would become so expansive that familiar subject-object distinctions would no longer be made. Hence, we have Peirce's doctrine that there will be no Secondness at the culmination of an infinite process of interpretation.

We have something of a paradox here. Objective standards are defined as standards that would be applied by members of the great community. But the state of harmony that defines the great community is possible only through an infinite process of moral inquiry and moral progress. For finite beings such as ourselves, such a perspective is unattainable; it is, as Royce admits, in this sense a lost cause. Further, the very notion of "objectivity," as we have here described it, is meaningless from the perspective of an inhabitant of the great community (since any perspective that arises within the great community will belong to it). "Objectivity," then, is an ideal for one who views the great community from a distance.

This leads us to a third point. Impartiality is not achievable for the finite human mind. It is a standard to which, insofar as we are moral beings, we aspire. Nevertheless, we are able to achieve shades of objectivity, and, to this extent, we can be impartial. When we speak of someone's judgment as being subjective, we generally imply that it is based on feelings, or merely personal standards. Subjective judgments are typical of those at the first level of moral life. As we approach the second level, we understand and choose the standards of a selected group, and our judgments are no longer so apt to reflect merely personal biases. To a degree, then, our judgments become less subjective and more objective. We are advancing morally, even if our natural loyalty is highly flawed. We are moving in the direction of the great community. At the third level, we consciously aspire toward the standards of the great community. As we achieve a modicum of success in this pursuit, our judgments become more objective, more impartial.

Fourth, the impartiality of which Royce speaks is not an absence of will or purpose and therefore cannot be confused with thoroughgoing forms of neutrality. It is the frame of reference from which all subordinate purposes are temporarily suspended for the sake of the supreme purpose—the highest moral purpose—which we have identified as the promotion of the interests of humanity. Royce's state of impartiality is, for instance, far less neutral than Descartes's state of doubt. Royce holds, with other pragmatists, that all thought is purposeful and therefore that thoroughgoing neutrality is impossible (in just the sense that reaching an endpoint to an infinite process of inquiry is impossible). More will be said on this matter, but, for now, let us return to our general discussion of the moral life.

Royce proclaims that morality begins with "the moral insight" that the will of one's neighbor is as real as one's own. His discussion of this insight is one of the cornerstones of his moral theory, and it warrants a thorough treatment. I will undertake this task in three stages. First, I will characterize the moral insight in a general way. Second, I will show how Royce's moral insight relates to similar insights by other philosophers—namely Plato, William James, John Stuart Mill, and Arthur Schopenhauer. Finally, I will discuss how the moral insight renders loyalty into a moral imperative.

THE MORAL INSIGHT

Royce believes that once we attain a genuine understanding of the will of our neighbor—where we are able temporarily to view his desires and his ideals as if they were our own—we will be struck with the insight that his will is as real as our own and therefore ought to be equally respected:

> Why is selfishness easier to me than unselfishness? Because it is easier for me to realize my own future, and my own desire about it, than to realize the desires of my neighbor. My will is the *datum*; his the dimly-conceived, remote fact. Hence it seems to me obvious that his will must be to me less significant than my own. (RAP, 147)

But if the root of selfishness is the contrast between the clarity of my own will and the vagueness of my neighbor's, then the solution to selfishness is a clear perception and understanding of the neighbor. If we are empathic enough to view the world through the eyes of our neighbor, then we will share his desires, and we will be privy to the plausibility of his ideals. The moral insight is an act of mediation in which we transgress the normal boundaries of our own perspective and find the common ground between ourselves and others.[4] Through this insight we understand that the neighbor's values ought to be respected as clearly as we see the need to embrace our own.

The plausibility of this conception is manifest upon reflection. For example, consider the frame of mind of a young woman who is viewing a movie such as *Butch Cassidy and the Sundance Kid*. From the opening scene, the film conveys the empathic viewer to another realm. She experiences the thrill of a train robbery, laughs with Etta as Butch shows off on his bicycle, cringes with fear as the main characters are assaulted with a barrage of gunfire. Quite readily, in an interval of a few minutes, our viewer provisionally acquires an alien set of values. She normally wants criminals to be captured and brought to justice, but now she wants these two to escape. She normally despises gambling and drinking but for now suspends those prejudices. Although certainly different from Butch and Sundance, our movie-goer is able to find common ground with these outlaws, not only sympathizing with them but, to a degree, understanding them. After the movie, as she returns to herself, she is apt to experience a kind of awakening. This event may consist of a fleeting sense of vertigo—the transient understanding that her own moral perspective is only one amongst several apparently viable alternatives. Or her response may take the form of a prolonged rumination. The experience may be pleasant or noxious, comforting or disturbing. But I would venture that all of us have experienced something like this at one time or another—if not in response to characters from a movie or a novel, then perhaps in response to the lives of family members, especially our children. It is a moment of moral insight.

What our viewer understands, perhaps vaguely, is that the values and enjoyments of Butch Cassidy and the Sundance Kid are self-legitimizing in the same way as her own. To truly understand these values is to esteem them. She realizes that if there is a moral absolute it must take the ideals of criminals, as well as her own ideals, into account. But there is more. The moviegoer has found that there is a connection between the values of others and her own, this manifested by the fact that she herself was able to understand and approve, however temporarily, the aims and ideals of Butch and Sundance. She comes to this realization because she has temporarily seen the world through their eyes. In this connectedness, the possibility for moral unity germinates.

This insight can be unpleasant for several reasons. First, it is apt to be a disruption. The thinker is awakened, as it were, from her dogmatic slumber. Moral beliefs that had become easy and regular are suddenly challenged. As Peirce might say, she is accosted by the irritation of doubt. Second, it is tragic. With the moral insight our vision of the moral universe is expanded, but also complicated. Though we have discovered a basis for moral unity, we also often find that the road to unity is impossibly long and arduous. Though we find strands of mutuality in foreign ideas, we realize how far these ideas ultimately are from our own—we realize that every attempt to formulate a unifying moral ideal will fall short. Outside of the perspective of an absolute being, the ability to mediate between conflicting values is limited. In other words, the moral insight facilitates our impartiality; it helps us bridge the gap between rival moral perspectives. But it also saddles us with a burgeoning set of moral ideals, and the knowledge that there can be no unifying theory, from our finite perspective, that is so comprehensive that it alleviates the anguish of conflicting moral commitments. This is a lesson that Royce illustrates in PL with the case of Robert E. Lee. It is the same lesson we learn from Sophocles' tragic protagonist, summarized in the following passage by MacIntyre:

> There are indeed crucial conflicts in which different virtues appear as making rival and incompatible claims upon us. But our situation is tragic in that we have to recognize the authority of both claims. There *is* an objective moral order, but our perceptions of it are such that we cannot bring rival moral truths into complete harmony with each other. . . . (AV, 143)

Sophocles' tragic protagonist, at least as understood by MacIntyre, experienced the moral insight. MacIntyre explains that the moral quandaries faced by such a protagonist are different from the ones faced by moral individualists such as Sartre, and it is worth a quick aside to see why. The tragic protagonist, let us say a missionary working against the odds in an alien and plague-ridden culture in Southeast Asia, is a woman who has overcome certain limitations that pertain to over-simplified and overly facile forms of morality. When discovering the hidden value in perspectives that were previously alien, the protagonist engages in a process of mediation, between her previous moral views and the alien ones. The moral principles that result from this process are significantly richer than her previous ones. Her devotion is more profound. She is able to express her moral ideal in manifold new ways and her exuberance seems more self-sustaining. Yet, because her commitments are more complicated, she also buys trouble. Unlike the moral simpleton, who sees everything in black and white, or the moral individualist, who everywhere sees incommensurability, our protagonist sees a vast connectedness of moral ideals, irreducible to a neat formula. Thus MacIntyre writes:

> One way in which the choice between rival goods in a tragic situation differs from the modern choice between incommensurable moral premises is that *both* of the alternative courses of action which confront the individual have to be recognized as leading to some authentic and substantial good. By choosing one I do nothing to diminish or derogate from the claim upon me of the other; and therefore, whatever I do, I shall have left undone what I ought to have done. (AV 224)

The pleasantness of the moral insight is also apparent in our summary of the tragic protagonist. There is comfort in the knowledge of the connectedness of moral values, however imperfect our conception of moral unity is doomed to be. And there is pleasure in the richness of the moral life that results from this insight.

In RUL, Royce identifies "the moral attitude" with reasonableness and impartiality.[5] It should not be difficult for the reader to see how this claim coheres with the position in RAP. Recall that we defined impartiality as the recognition that all desires, impulses, and ideals are values that are, prima facie, worthy of respect. Through the moral insight, we become more impartial as we recognize the validity of objective standards as well as the impossibility that we will ever adequately formulate them. Everyone has applied objective standards, however imperfectly. With the moral insight we come closer to understanding them and should consequently improve our capacity to employ them.

Many of the above points will become clearer if we compare Royce's moral insight with similar insights of other philosophers.

Moral Insight in Plato, James, Mill, and Schopenhauer

In *Symposium*, Plato gives a five-step account of moral development. Through Socrates, who is relating the lessons he learned from Diotima, Plato details how one who begins with the love of physical beauty may ascend to the heights of wisdom:

Well then, she began, the candidate for this initiation cannot, if his efforts are to be rewarded, begin too early to devote
himself to the beauties of the body. First of all, if his preceptor
instructs him as he should, he will fall in love with the beauty of
one individual body, so that his passion may give life to noble
discourse. Next, he must consider how nearly related the beauty
of any one body is to the beauty of any other, when he will see
that if he is to devote himself to loveliness of form it will be absurd to deny that the beauty of each and every body is the same.
Having reached this point, he must set himself to be the lover of
every lovely body, and bring his passion for the one into due proportion by deeming it of little or of no importance.

Next he must grasp that the beauties of the body are as nothing to the beauties of the soul, so that wherever he meets with
spiritual loveliness, even in the husk of an unlovely body, he will
find it beautiful enough to fall in love with and cherish—and
beautiful enough to quicken in his heart a longing for such discourse as tends toward the building of a noble nature. And from
this he will be led to contemplate the beauty of laws and institutions. And when he discovers how nearly every kind of beauty is
akin to every other he will conclude that the beauty of the body
is not, after all, of so great moment.

And next, his attention should be diverted from institutions
to the sciences, so that he may know the beauty of every kind of
knowledge. And thus, by scanning beauty's wide horizon, he will
be saved from a slavish and illiberal devotion to the individual
loveliness of a single boy, a single man, or a single institution.
And, turning his eyes toward the open sea of beauty, he will find
in such contemplation the seed of the most fruitful discourse and
the loftiest thought, and reap a golden harvest of philosophy,
until, confirmed and strengthened, he will come upon one single
form of knowledge, the knowledge of the beauty I am about to
speak of. (Plato 1961, 561–562)

Similarities with Royce are evident. The first step—the "love" of the
beauty of an individual body—is a crude and typical entry into social life.
The individual at this stage is like the infant who views his mother as an

automated provider of services. He is enthralled with a social object, but his cognizance of the inner life of this object is extremely vague. His appreciation of the beloved is subjective and essentially selfish.

At the next level, the individual apprehends the characteristics of the beloved in other objects. His social universe is expanded. Though the individual still estimates the worth of social objects from the standpoint of his own selfish interests, he nevertheless begins to understand that they have something—apart from his interest in them—in common. In this insight, his powers of abstraction are born. There are two important parallels with Royce. First, Plato and Royce both think that the recognition of similarities between diverse social objects, in whatever crude or inadequate form it initially appears, is an essential early step in moral development. In Royce's account, this recognition is generally described as the result of a comparison of these objects with one's self. In Plato, the objects are compared with each other. Both types of comparison are no doubt operative early in the life of any child, and the difference of emphasis between the two thinkers should not be allowed to obscure the similarities. Second, it is worth noting that both thinkers associate progress in moral development with progress in intellectual development. Recall that Royce considers both reasonableness and impartiality to be prerequisites of any substantial moral insight. The power of abstraction here chronicled by Plato is part of what he had in mind.

Out of the power of abstraction comes the capacity for impartiality. Viewing social objects as bearers of important common characteristics helps the individual to detach himself from his particular passion for the first beloved individual and cultivate a passion for the universal (though it be conceived at this point rather dimly), or at least for the whole collection of individuals who exhibit the universal. This detachment constitutes the third step of development. Though the individual at this stage may still be thought of as selfish, he is also apt to be a self-denying self in just the sense that Kierkegaard's "A" is. In fact, throughout Plato's entire account, there is an overtone of such aestheticism, constituted not only by the fact that Plato chooses beauty as the primary object of the fledgling moralist, but also by the fact that the individual always stands so radically apart from this object. Recall the difference in emphasis between Plato and Royce on the primary path by which individuals develop their powers of abstraction. Plato's student of morals loses himself because he never relates the object of devotion back to himself. Of course, the importance of Plato's third step, for Royce, would lie in the cultivation of impartiality.

At the fourth stage, the individual discovers forms of beauty other than physical beauty and finds that they are superior. Plato introduces the notion of "spiritual loveliness." It is an unresolved matter whether and how beauty of the spirit is anything other than analogous to physical beauty. One is tempted to side with Mill and understand spiritual beauty as related to physical beauty in that both are enjoyed. To some degree at least, Plato seems to endorse the idea that our appreciation for higher objects is conditioned by pleasure. But, with Aristotle and Royce, Plato is more accurately portrayed as holding (1) that the philosopher is one who by nature desires knowledge, (2) that the understanding of certain objects imparts a fuller and more comprehensive form of knowledge than the understanding of others, (3) that it is on the basis of this comprehensiveness that the former objects are classified as "higher," and (4) that the greater pleasure we feel through the apprehension of higher objects is complementary, rather than constituting the moral worth of knowledge. For Royce, the moral insight facilitates our recognition of the varying degrees of fitness of moral objects (i.e., of causes). The greater our ability to comprehend the inner life of others, the more accurately we are able to understand which values permeate human life. These values are the higher ideals, the greater causes. Collective ideals—the ideals of communities—are, of course, the ones Royce esteems the highest. They are unifying. They are the ideals that facilitate the moral striving for comprehensiveness.

The fifth step in moral progress is an extension of the fourth. Here, the objects of science are added to the repertoire of the aspirant. Plato's moral vision is finally completed by "one single form of knowledge," comprehending all that is knowable. Diotima goes on to express this knowledge in words compatible with Plato's general account of the knowledge of a Form—knowledge that is purely intellectual, entirely divorced from its corporeal roots. Here we find an important basis of disagreement between Plato and Royce.

The difficulty with Plato's account of the moral insight stems from his lack of acknowledgment of what the mind contributes to the nature and worthiness of its ideals. One of the fundamental aspects of Royce's moral insight is the fact that human desires and values are claims that establish—*for themselves*—their own prima facie validity. Whatever the nature of moral perfection, it will be a perfection, at least in part, because it is a state of affairs that responds to these desires and values. For Plato, the ideal moral unity stands apart from human striving, something wholly external, fixed and complete, a *telos* isolated from its pursuers.

One of the implications of Plato's view is that the Good may be appreciated by someone in a state of isolation. Social influences are important in order that we be steered in the direction of the Good, not because they are a necessary part of our final appreciation of moral perfection (thus, Socrates' self-description as a midwife). Social life, at the final stage of moral development, is abandoned for the moral reclusiveness of one who dwells entirely in private thought.[6] For Royce, the *telos*—the great community—is an embodiment of the absolute and is wholly understood only from the perspective of the absolute. From this perspective it is indeed fixed and complete. But the fixity and completeness that are apparent to the absolute, as history is viewed *totem simul*, are inaccessible to finite creatures, who can only view the *telos* as the result of an infinitude of progress, as something achieved, and achieved socially, not given.

Let us turn our attention to Royce's best friend and colleague at Harvard, William James. In "The Moral Philosopher and the Moral Life," James gives an account of moral insight that is clearly influenced by Royce's notion.[7] He begins by differentiating between three questions that are relevant to ethics:

> Let them be called respectively the *psychological* question, the *metaphysical* question, and the *casuistic* question. The psychological question asks after the historical *origin* of our moral ideas and judgments; the metaphysical question asks what the very *meaning* of the words 'good,' 'ill,' and 'obligation' are; the casuistic question asks what is the *measure* of the various goods and ills which men recognize, so that the philosopher may settle the true order of human obligations. (James [1967] 1977, 611)

James is less interested in the psychological question in this essay than he is in the other two, and we will pass this question over entirely except for the following comment. James traces a far greater portion of our moral ideas and judgments to "purely inward forces" of individuals than Royce does. James writes that "All the higher, more penetrating ideals are revolutionary. They present themselves far less in the guise of effects of past experience than in that of probable causes of future experience (James [1967] 1977, 613). Royce, on the other hand, believes that moral theorists, though occasionally propelled by a spark of genuine spontaneity, are generally best characterized as clarifying ideas already present in the substratum of the moral activities of their culture (SMP 8–9). As we have discussed, Royce thinks that revolutionary ideals are inherently conservative. It is interesting that Royce occupies a middle ground on this issue between James and Dewey, far more appreciative of social influences than James, but significantly more removed from social determinism than Dewey.

James begins his discussion of the metaphysical question by noting that words with moral import would have no application in a purely physical universe. The situation is different if we introduce a single sentient being:

> The moment one sentient being, however, is made a part of the universe, there is a chance for goods and evils really to exist. Moral relations now have their *status*, in that being's consciousness. So far as he feels anything to be good, he *makes* it good. It *is* good, for him; and being good from him, is absolutely good, for he is the sole creator of values in that universe, and outside of his opinion things have no moral character at all. (James [1967] 1977, 615)

James here isolates two important aspects of the moral insight: that values arise in the context of consciousness and that each value is self-legitimizing in a prima facie sense. James remarks that the solitary thinker will have to arrange his values hierarchically, since they are bound at times to conflict. Thus, even at this level, the authority of moral ideals is subject to mediation by other ideals.

If we enter another thinker, James points out that several possibilities pertain. First, the thinkers could wholly ignore one another's values. In such a case, the universe would be rendered into a moral dualism, devoid of unity. Each thinker would wholly lack moral insight about the condition of the other and would proceed as if a solitary sentient being.

There is a second possibility, contingent, as James declares, on one or more of the thinkers adopting values that animate the moral philosopher. One of the thinkers could recognize for both what was previously recognized only for himself—that each value establishes, for itself, a degree of legitimacy.

> But the moment we take a steady look at the question, *we see not only that without a claim actually made by some concrete person there can be no obligation, but that there is some obligation wherever there is a claim.* Claim and obligation are, in fact, coextensive terms; they cover each other exactly. (James [1967] 1977, 617)

James specifies two commitments of moral philosophers that underlie this understanding: (1) impartiality, and (2) the desire for unity. It is impartiality, coupled with a power of empathy, that allows a thinker to view a second thinker in the way that James views the solitary sentient being. On this point Royce surely would agree. With the desire for unity, this insight leads to an effort to establish an inclusive collective ideal. How to implement such an ideal is the *casuistic* question.

One of the key differences between Royce and James is in their accounts of the desire for unity. For Royce, the desire for social unity abides in the heart of each human being. But, though present in each of us, it becomes fully conscious only through the moral insight. James—at least in "The Moral Philosopher and the Moral Life"—portrays the desire for unity as an arbitrary personal addition of the thinker, coming to fruition wholly apart from the moral insight. That is, for James the moral insight is an apprehension of the hypothetical imperative that *given we desire an impartial, unifying moral ideal* then we ought to respect every valuation of each sentient being. For Royce, the moral insight, at least in its highest form, is the more comprehensive understanding that the valuations of each human being[8] are similar to our own and thus ought to be respected, not merely because they are self-legitimizing on an individual basis (though this is a factor) but also because they express a degree of underlying unity between their bearers and all humanity. Ultimately, Royce believes that what James describes as a hypothetical imperative is actually a categorical imperative, because all moral agents will a unifying moral ideal.[9] This is not to say that Royce thinks that everyone wills or desires the same things—hopefully we have already dispatched such an interpretation. Royce thinks there is a real conflict of human aims and that this conflict is not resolved by the moral insight alone (if it were, we would not need God). However, there is, according to Royce, a universal desire for harmony, and it comes to fruition in the moral insight.

On the issue of the desire for unity, both James and Royce seem to offer plausible accounts. I doubt their differences could be resolved on any straightforward empirical basis, given the unlikelihood of establishing criteria for identifying a latent desire for harmony. Ultimately one would have to examine James's and Royce's respective metaphysical doctrines. Such a task is beyond our scope. Nevertheless, I submit that James is astray of Royce's moral insight at least in part because he is hampered by a naïve conception of moral perfection. This naïveté contributes to his failure to appreciate the connectedness of moral ideals. James writes that

> If the ethical philosopher were only asking after the best *imaginable* system of goods he would indeed have an easy task; for all demands as such are *primâ facie* respectable, and the best simply imaginary world would be one in which every demand was gratified as soon as made. (James [1967] 1977, 621)

But James is surely wrong. It is not difficult to see that a world in which every demand were immediately met, every desire immediately quenched, would be tedious beyond imagination.[10] Later in "The Moral Philosopher and the Moral Life," James speaks of the difference between the easygoing and the strenuous mood. It is doubtful that even the most easygoing would be happy with a life of pure, effortless satisfaction; but those of the strenuous mood would certainly not be. The advice of Theodore Roosevelt still casts a spell; it echoes in the lives of Gandhi and Rommel:

> I wish to preach, not a doctrine of ignoble ease, but the doctrine of the strenuous life, the life of toil and effort, of labor and strife; to preach that highest form of success which comes, not to the man who desires mere easy peace, but to the man who does not shrink from danger, from hardship, or from bitter toil, and who out of these wins the splendid ultimate triumph. (Roosevelt 1900, 1)

Royce, though he was personally no fan of Roosevelt, would heartily agree.

An implication of James's belief that moral perfection consists in the immediate fulfillment of all desires is the position that the universe is ineradicably morally deficient. Both Royce and James agree that if moral unity is a legitimate cause, it is nevertheless infinitely distant. But one who believes, with James, that delaying gratification is morally undesirable could never hold that the quest for moral unity is the supreme end of a human life. There are too many obstacles. Thus, James's moral insight has implications different from Royce's. Royce's glimpse of partial unity spurs him to a quest for more unity. When he sees it is possible to mediate between divergent values, he takes up the mantle of mediation. In this regard, Royce is, once again, closer to Mill than he is to James.[11] James, on the other hand, never views the thoroughgoing pursuit of unity as a legitimate option. He is everywhere impressed with the divergence of moral values. The magnitude of this divergence for James is enough to convince him of its ineradicability. James claims that "various ideals have no common character apart from the fact that they are ideals." Royce stands in utter contrast, claiming that part of the moral insight is the realization that humans are similar in manifold, and perhaps poorly understood, ways, that their inner lives are similar, and that their diverging ideals spring from similar ultimate purposes.

James finishes his essay with a look at the role of God:

> It would seem, too,— and this is my final conclusion,— that the stable and systematic moral universe for which the ethical philosopher asks is fully possible only in a world where there is a divine thinker with all-enveloping demands. (628)

For James, the existence of such a thinker would have to be a postulate. For Royce, there is good evidence for such a belief, some of which is grounded in the moral insight.[12] "The Moral Philosopher and the Moral Life" was first published in 1891—six years after *The Religious Aspect of Philosophy*. James credits this latter work with setting forth the ethical role of God "with great freshness and force." In the end, however, James does not recognize the full force of Royce's account of the moral insight.

James's account of the moral insight leads to a distinctly utilitarian answer to the casuistic question. As we have remarked, Royce is certainly no utilitarian. Though we will not cover James's discussion of his utilitarian ideal, I would like to briefly remark on how another utilitarian, John Stuart Mill, gives a distinctly more Roycean account of the moral insight than James's version. Mill occupies a middle ground when he remarks that "The social state is at once so natural, so necessary, and so habitual to man, that except in some unusual circumstances or by an effort of voluntary abstraction, he never conceives himself otherwise than as a member of a body; and this association is riveted more and more, as mankind are further removed from the state of savage independence" (Mill [1861] 1957, 40).

With Royce, Mill recognizes the centrality of social elements of human character. James's notion of a solitary sentient being would be, for Mill, a "voluntary abstraction," of the sort noted above—of limited usefulness to one who aspires to give a comprehensive account of human moral life. Further, Mill recognizes, with Royce, that there is a moral insight that not only is stimulated by a desire for unity but that augments this desire by enhancing the individual's understanding of (1) the degree to which such a unity is already present and (2) the means by which it may be increased. For Mill, this moral insight consists of the attitude that human beings are equal and the realization that "society between human beings . . . is manifestly impossible on any other footing than that the interests of all are to be consulted." Mill describes, through his discussion of this moral insight, the psychological basis for a sentiment that is very close to that of Royce's loyalist:

> They [people who grow up in more advanced societies] are also familiar with the fact of co-operating with others and proposing to themselves a collective, not an individual, interest as the aim (at least for the time being) of their actions. So long as they are co-operating, their ends are identified with those of others; there is at least a temporary feeling that the interests of others are their own interests. (Mill [1861] 1957, 41)

Mill departs from Royce and sides with James in that he ultimately relates even the most unifying tendencies back to individuals for whom the untutored state is one of "savage independence." While Royce holds that social conceptions are as primordial as individualistic ones, the other thinkers characterize the primordial state of nature as one where humans view themselves as isolated beings with isolated interests. Mill's misgivings about abstracting the individuals from their social context notwithstanding, he seems to hold that the human being is first of all an individual and develops socially only through the influence of contingent social forces. Royce, in contrast, maintains that it is no more possible to be an individual outside a social context than it is to be a member of society without being an individual. Mill's tendency to isolate the individual is no doubt the result of his exposure to the empirical psychology, harshly criticized by Royce, that begins its examination of the human psyche with an account of isolated sense perceptions—assuming that sense perceptions could be experienced as discrete events apart from some process of social conditioning. Only under the influence of such a psychology would it be possible for Mill to develop his account of the human good in terms of pleasure and the absence of pain.

We have already spoken of Schopenhauer's philosophy in our discussion of the ideal of the self-denying self. Of course, Schopenhauer's moral ideal arises out of his version of the moral insight. This relation is summarized in the following passage:

> Now if, as a rare exception, we come across a man who possesses a considerable income, but uses only a little of it for himself, and gives all the rest to persons in distress, whilst he himself forgoes many pleasures and comforts, and we try to make clear to ourselves the action of this man, we shall find, quite apart from the dogmas by which he himself will make his action intelligible to his faculty of reason, the simplest general expression and the essential character of his way of acting to be that he *makes less distinction than is usually made between himself and others. . . .* The *principium individuationis*, the form of the phenomenon, no longer holds him so firmly in its grasp, but the suffering he sees in others touches him almost as closely as does his own. He therefore tries to strike a balance between the two, denies himself pleasures, undergoes privations, in order to alleviate another's suffering. He perceives that the distinction between himself and others, which to the wicked man is so great a gulf, belongs only to a fleeting, deceptive phenomenon. He recognizes immediately,

and without reasons or arguments, that the in-itself of his own
phenomenon is also that of others. . . . (Schopenhauer [1958]
1969 I, 372)

This could be Royce speaking, except that (1) the perception of the inner
life of others is here portrayed as being of the nature of a feeling—of sympathy—rather than, as per Royce, of thought—of empathy—which includes both feeling and cognition (RAP 154), and (2) the unity of which
Schopenhauer speaks differs in important ways from Royce's sense of
unity. For Schopenhauer, we are all manifestations of a single thing-in-
itself, and we are thus, ultimately, not individuals at all. For Royce, our
individuality is a metaphysical fact, which stands alongside our unity. It is
a common ideal that provides unity in Royce's case. For Schopenhauer, as
we have seen, there is no common aim or ideal—only desire and suffering are shared.

We have commented that Schopenhauer's rejection of unifying ideals
leads to his pessimism. It is worth remarking that the rationale for rejecting a unifying ideal, in Schopenhauer, is always based on the same kind
of view of the morally perfect world that we have criticized in James.
Schopenhauer consistently views struggle and suffering as evidence of the
world's imperfection. Royce, we have seen, differs. In *The Spirit of Modern Philosophy*, Royce criticizes Schopenhauer on exactly this point,
sounding a lot like Roosevelt: "The spirit exists by accepting and by tri-
umphing over the tragedy of the world. Restlessness, longing, grief,—
these are evils, fatal evils, and they are everywhere in the world; but the
spirit must be strong enough to endure them. In this strength is the solution. And, after all, it is just endurance that is the essence of spirituality"
(SMP 263).

Royce's mature conception of the moral insight results in his mature
version of genuine loyalty—as we will shortly see. Likewise, the accounts
of moral insight that we find in other thinkers also result in moral ideals.
For instance, Plato's version yields a distinctly Platonic ideal.[13] The ideals
of Plato, James, and Mill do not correspond nicely to any of the four
moral ideals we discussed in chapter 2. No doubt, there are strong elements in Plato of the heroic ideal. These elements are expressed, for example, in his respect for statesmanship and courage in battle and in his
view that moral virtue and happiness are inextricably linked. But Plato, in

his notion of higher and lower passions, and his ultimate disavowal of the latter, is also close kin to the self-denying self. James is in many ways a rebel, but tempers the rebel's disregard for social harmony. Mill, as we have seen, expresses an ideal that in many respects approximates Royce's, but also differs from Royce on crucial issues. Royce would no doubt argue that none of these ideals resolves the paradox of self-realization except as it approximates the spirit of loyalty. Neither Plato nor Mill nor James is able, in Royce's view, to satisfy the psychological need for loyalty. Further, the theories of these thinkers are ethically vulnerable based on deficiencies in the moral insight from which they proceed. These deficiencies we have already discussed.

Royce's four ideals, discussed in chapter 2, were chosen, no doubt, not to constitute an exhaustive list but because they collectively cover more territory than any four comparable ideals. Though there are many viable moral ideals that do not fit neatly into one of these four categories, virtually all the salient general characteristics of the diverging ideals are found somewhere within the nexus of the four ideals chosen by Royce.[14]

Before we move on to our discussion of how Royce expresses his moral insight in the ideal of loyalty, I would briefly like to address a minor problem. This problem can be formulated by looking at the hero. The hero is one who lives at the first moral level. He is essentially selfish, this selfishness manifested by the fact that he cannot see his life as a success except in the circumstance that he is the recipient of fame, riches, power, or some other aspect of good fortune. It would seem that such an individual lacked any semblance of the moral insight described by Royce. It is, then, not surprising that Royce often writes as if what I have identified as the first level of moral life is premoral. This position certainly seems to be the one that he adopts in RAP. If the moral life begins with the moral insight, such a view seems necessary. Yet, in RUL, Royce refers to the first level as "moral." This would seem to be an inconsistency. Perhaps it is. But, I will argue, only a minor one. To understand why, it is helpful to recall the theory of interpretation.

My own life, according to this theory, is a collection of thought-signs, intimately related along a linear, temporal continuum. Likewise, my community is a collection of thought-signs, related by common ideals. Finally, the universe is a still larger collection of thought-signs. Now suppose I were to live each moment in isolation, disconnected from the moment before, with no memory and no ability to anticipate the future. In this state, the life of prudence would be impossible. Comprehensive ideals of any kind would be inconceivable. Each act would transpire as if it were my first and last. My life would accurately reflect what Royce has called "a solipsism of the present moment."

Then suppose I became endowed with a perfect memory and a profound perspective on my future and how it could be shaped by my present decisions. This insight would transform my existence. No longer would I act on every momentary impulse. I would learn to order my activities so that both present and future fulfillments were maximized. In essence, I would learn to respect my future desires as equals of my present ones. But this idea is a species of moral insight. The moral insight occurs when we are able to appreciate thought-signs that are not our own. It seems reasonable to view the insight as a three-stage process, occurring as we successively cultivate three abilities: (1) the ability to appreciate our own past and future thought-signs, (2) the ability to appreciate the thought-signs of those who are closely related to us, and (3) the ability to appreciate the thought-signs of all human beings.[15] Of course, to appreciate a thought-sign, in the sense intended, is to interpret it accurately. The will to interpret becomes the spark that ignites the moral life. In fact, the will to interpret covers the same ground for the later Royce what the will for harmony does for the early Royce.

The hero, then, along with others who dwell at the first level of moral life (Epicureans, for instance), is a moral being just insofar as he approximates the moral insight. His moral insight is relatively dim, consisting mostly of his ability to appreciate his own past and future thought-signs. It is likely that he has much to learn about the inner life of others and how that inner life is connected to his own. Nevertheless, because he is able to evaluate impartially and prioritize his own present and future desires and satisfactions, he is able to formulate a plan. This ability, we have seen, qualifies him as a moral being. His shortcomings, on the other hand, ensure that his moral life will not measure up to the highest standard, unless he develops a more profound moral insight.

LOYALTY TO LOYALTY

We have thus far in this chapter advanced two claims: (1) each human being has a need to be loyal (this need being grounded in his or her need to establish a satisfying personal identity), and (2) each human being ought to respect the needs of all other human beings equally, alongside his or her own (this obligation being grounded in the moral insight). Once we accept these two claims, it follows that we ought to respect both our own and our neighbor's need for loyalty. This means, for Royce, that we should try to cultivate a form of personal loyalty that will harmonize, as much as possible, with the loyalties of others. Further, we should seek to augment the loyalties of others, just as we should strive to strengthen our own. This harmonious growth of loyalties is the highest cause for each of us. When we devote ourselves to this cause we are loyal to loyalty. For Royce, loyalty to loyalty is our highest moral obligation:

> In so far as it lies in your power, so choose your cause and so serve it, that, by reason of your choice and of your service, there shall be more loyalty in the world rather than less. And, in fact so choose and so serve your individual cause as to secure thereby the greatest possible increase of loyalty amongst men. More briefly: *In choosing and in serving the cause to which you are to be loyal, be, in any case, loyal to loyalty.* (PL 57)

We have described loyalty as devotion to the well-being of a community. Loyalty to loyalty is devotion to the well-being of a community that defines itself by the commitment to strong and harmonious loyalties. In HGC, this is how Royce conceives the great community. Thus, loyalty to loyalty can be conceived as loyalty to the great community.

There is, however, a second way of conceiving the great community that appears in Royce—as a fully realized community of interpretation, akin to what we find in Peirce (PC 389). I will refer to this conception (which we briefly mentioned earlier) as the metaphysical conception of the great community. In HGC, the great community is viewed from the perspective of the present. In the metaphysical conception, it is viewed from the perspective of infinitude. Though I would argue that the two perspectives can be reconciled, that problem is not my concern here. My interest in this matter is twofold: (1) I wish to avert confusion about the two alternative formulations, and (2) I wish to urge the reader to accept the former formulation—let us call it the moral formulation of the great community—as a more central aspect of Royce's moral program.

As we commented earlier, the final achievement reflected in the meta-physical conception of the great community occurs only as history is viewed *totum simul*, from the infinite perspective of God. Three reasons explain why I think that such a conception is less valuable for moral pur-poses than one in which the great community is associated with a quest to harmonize and intensify loyalties. First, it is not at all clear that loyalty would be possible after an infinite process of moral growth, since pre-sumably there would be no unrealized causes. Royce has described the moral life as a life of struggle, but, once again, it is not clear that such a life is possible after the culmination of all struggles. Thus, if loyalty to the great community is conceived as loyalty to an infinitely distant state of harmony, then it is not the same as loyalty to loyalty. Instead, it would be loyalty to a state of affairs in which the need for loyalty has been eradi-cated—an ideal strangely similar to Schopenhauer's.[16] The notion of loy-alty loses its ethical centrality from such a perspective.[17]

Second, the great community is conceptually more accessible when it is viewed as a community of mutually complementary loyalties than when it is conceived as a state of wholly realized causes. As we have noted al-ready, it is not clear how individuals would differentiate themselves in the inevitable state of psychological transparency that would characterize the latter community. Such a world is an abstraction, remote from our own, and not likely to be a very useful cause for devotees who must make dif-ficult moral decisions.

Third, the notion of loyalty to the moral conception of the great community leaves room for the notion of competition. To clarify, let us distinguish between two forms of competition: (1) destructive competi-tion, during which one aims at annihilating the competitor, and (2) con-structive competition, during which one aims at the improvement of both self and competitor. An example of the first is warfare. An example of the second is sparring, as it generally occurs within a *karate dojo*. Construc-tive competition is not merely morally acceptable; it is one of the corner-stones of moral development. Royce writes at length about it in his dis-cussion of training for loyalty. But in a community where every cause is realized, competition of any kind would seem to be excluded.

Fourth, and perhaps most important, remember that loyalty is a virtue. For Royce, as for Aristotle, virtuous action should not merely aim at an external goal but also be an end in itself. Loyal action that aims at loyalty is just such an end in itself. Such loyalty to loyalty, as we have seen, is equated with loyalty to the moral conception of the great community, not to the metaphysical conception. From a purely practical point of view, loyalty to excessively remote goals tends to be unsatisfying. George Leonard, in his book *Mastery*, a very readable account of the journey to excellence, documents how individuals who do not experience a degree of fulfillment at their current level of development are apt to abandon the quest for excellence. He argues that, if we are to progress, we must not only be motivated to achieve technically higher levels of virtue but also to feel pleasure in our current practice. He characterizes the life of the master as one composed of brief spurts of learning or improvement, followed by long plateaus where one is apparently fixed at a single level of achievement. If we do not develop a love for the plateau, Leonard argues, we will never progress. Instead we will become dabblers, moving from one cause to another. Similar reasoning occurs in Royce, who states that "Fickleness is the most dangerous foe of the art of loyalty" (RPL II, 46).

Genuine loyalty, then, is best conceived as loyalty to loyalty, and loyalty to loyalty can be equated with loyalty to a community defined by the ideal of cultivating and harmonizing loyalties. Several misunderstandings are apt to occur at this point and should be avoided at the outset. First, the doctrine of loyalty to loyalty is *not* a new form of utilitarianism, where the moral worth of an act depends wholly on whether or not it has the end result of maximizing loyalty. Royce, like Kant, resolutely and consistently locates the source of moral worth in the will of moral agents. Good actions are loyal actions. An action performed out of greed or hatred is not a loyal action. Such an act may have the end result of cultivating loyalty, but that does not, for Royce, make it a good action.[18] With Aristotle and other virtue ethicists, Royce would hold that the spirit of loyalty is expressed more frequently in actions proceeding from habit—reflecting the character of the moral agent—than it is in actions proceeding immediately from deliberation about the maximization of loyalty. For Royce, the intention to promote loyalty informs our habits and becomes part of our character. Royce further distinguishes himself from the utilitarians by refusing to view loyalty as something analogous to happiness or pleasure; loyalty is not possessed by the individual, in the sense that one can possess happiness, but is, rather, a thoroughly moral relation between the individual and a community. Royce, however, does not wholly side with

Kant against the utilitarians. He judges the ultimate value of a moral ideal—of a cause—by the extent to which it promotes loyalty generally, that is, by its results.

Second, Royce omits the technical discussion of reasonableness and impartiality in PL, and the critical reader is apt to conclude that he is guilty of the same fallacy as Mill, namely, deriving a statement containing an *ought* from one that contains only the nonmoral *is*. Royce insists that such a transition is impossible—that morality is the offspring of the moral insight—but, unfortunately, he does not make this view explicit in PL. Perhaps he is playing to the lack of sophistication of the general audience to which PL is addressed, expecting that the more critical readers of PL will recall the arguments of RAP. In any case, Royce believes that the highest level of moral life commences with an understanding of the connectedness of ideals, where enlightened selfishness gives way to a universal, outwardly focused form of loyalty that is at once the highest good for the individual and for humanity. This is not to say that selfish interests are best served by altruistic behavior, but rather that, with genuine insight, the outlook of the moral agent is transformed; his ideals are no longer selfish.[19] In these matters Royce is close to Kant. Both insist that higher moral principles comprise a specific realm of objects of the rational intellect. Unlike Kant, Royce exposes how this moral realm is connected, metaphysically and psychologically, to other realms of thought, and how all intelligent thought is, in some degree, moral.[20]

Royce, then, with Kant and Dewey, believes that "ought" statements are always also "is" statements, or are initially connected with "is" statements. "Ought," for these thinkers, is created by the will of moral agents. "Ought" statements that are categorical rather than merely hypothetical imperatives arise when we are compelled to recognize an ideal merely by virtue of the fact that we are moral agents. In Royce's case, the moral agent is conceived first of all as one who wills to be a self. The will to be a self begets a need for loyalty. This need, combined with the capacity to perceive the same need in his or her fellows, is the precondition of moral agency for Royce. As we have seen, the moral agent, so conceived, is compelled to recognize the ideal of universal loyalty. All further moral obligations will result from the moral agent's individual response to this imperative, coupled with the contingencies of the agent's life experience. When we commit ourselves to an ideal, we take on manifold obligations.

The commitment and the obligations it engenders are as real a part of the universe as any other aspect of our inner lives. In essence, the Roycean moral agent says: "This much *is* the case: I need and will, above all else, to be loyal. I recognize this need in others, and my recognition of this need in others leads me to will that their causes also be realized, along with my own. Devotion to this end—this loyalty to loyalty—I experience as a firm, overarching, and inescapable commitment. From this I conclude that I *ought* to be loyal to loyalty, because no other source of moral obligation is possible for one such as I."[21]

With John Dewey, Royce believes that sharp divisions between moral and nonmoral realms of life result in false dualisms and bad metaphysics. Ultimately, for Royce, to live a totally nonmoral life would be to live a life of total isolation—isolated in time from oneself and isolated from others. But to live in this way would be not to live at all; it would be not to exist.[22]

A third possible misunderstanding is related to the second. One is apt to be confused by Royce's statement that "In loyalty, when loyalty is properly defined, is the fulfillment of the whole moral law" (PL, 9). This is not the claim that loyalty is the only moral principle and that the others are derivable from the notion of loyalty. Rather, it is the claim that a full-bodied notion of loyalty will incorporate moral principles—such as the principle of impartiality and the principle of autonomy—that are extrinsic to loyalty as it occurs naturally. Royce's original definition of loyalty—the willing and practical and thoroughgoing devotion of a self to a cause—is a definition of natural loyalty. The imperative to be loyal in this sense is not a summation of the whole moral law. For Royce, as he expresses himself in PL, loyalty "properly defined" is the love of the great community. This conception emerges when one who has discovered natural loyalty becomes endowed with the spirit of impartiality. Fully comprehended in that sense, loyalty is a synthesis of the principle of natural loyalty with the principle of impartiality. As Royce made clear in his later years, it is also a synthesis of the three leading ideas of ethics: autonomy, goodness, and duty.

Avoiding the caveats here indicated, Royce's notion of loyalty to loyalty seems to be the moral ideal we have sought. It now remains to return to the world of medicine and study how Royce would conceive the loyal physician.

5

❖

The Physician-Patient Relation

We have established that moral beings—including physicians—have a moral and psychological need to serve a cause. The morally mature person recognizes that he is not alone, not independent, but is, and has been from the moment of birth, part of a community. He has freely chosen one or more natural communities to serve and cherish and is joined in this endeavor by fellow members of these communities, all viewing the same past and future events as part of their collective life. His selfhood is expansive; his life includes the lives of these others.

Further, he has learned that the communities he loyally serves are related to other communities, themselves peopled by loyal servants, and that his devotion is related to theirs. He thinks of his natural communities as contributors to a future great community, which includes all of these communities, all of humanity. Insofar as he is able to visualize this ideal, he unites all the various competing values in an all-inclusive perspective. Every human experience becomes part of a single moral life. He may be a physician. If so, of what does his loyalty consist?

We will begin our examination of this question in this chapter by looking at loyalty between physicians and patients. First, we will seek to understand the sense in which the physician-patient relation constitutes a community and about the characteristics of this community. We will note two characteristics of great importance: (1) the community of physician and patient, conceived purely as a dyad, engenders a degenerate cause, incompatible with true loyalty, and (2) as such a dyad, this community is unstable. This instability will become clear as we examine the faultiness of a model of the physician-patient relation that portrays it in just such dyadic terms—the entrepreneurial model. Second, we will search for a means of purging this instability and find that our solution, theoretically speaking, is to situate the physician and patient within a triadic social structure. In practice, we will find, this means that both physician and patient are members of a "greater medical community," which commands the loyalty of both and which mediates the actual and potential tensions within their relationship. We will consider the characteristics of this community at some length. Third, we will briefly examine how each of the three species of loyalty—which Royce derived from the model of the family—are important to the physician-patient relation. We will conclude by discussing how our triadic account of clinical medicine affects our conception of professional ethics.

Physician and Patient

When one asks to whom or to what the physician should be loyal, the rather obvious response is "To patients!" This response can be taken in one of at least three ways: the physician ought to be loyal to (1) the therapeutic community that includes the physician as the therapist and any single patient with whom the physician is presently engaged; or (2) to the therapeutic community that includes the physician as the therapist and all the physician's patients; or (3) to the potential therapeutic community that includes the physician as the therapist and all actual and prospective patients. In this section I will consider the first of these alternatives.

I will refer to the social group that consists of a single therapist and a single patient as the "clinical dyad." Loyalty, we recall, is devotion to the interests or ideals of a community. But is the dyad a community? I would say yes.

Both the physician and the patient hold certain events to be important, and they organize their relationship around these events. There is, first, the events comprising the patient's constellation of symptoms or worries. As we will see, these events are viewed somewhat differently by patient and physician, but both seek to interpret the same events. Then, there is a common hope or expectation—relief for the patient. Thus, we can classify the physician-patient relationship as a community of memory and a community of expectation.[1]

What, then, are the interests of the clinical dyad? Answers to questions about the interests of a community often hinge on considerations about the origins of the community. We could ask: What are the circumstances under which this community came into existence? or, For what purpose are these persons associated? Alternatively, one might seek to discover the interests of the clinical dyad through examining its functional apparatus—How do things transpire within the context of this community? We will consider each of these questions.[2]

A precondition for the existence of a clinical dyad is the fact that people get sick and they get injured. (For our purposes, I will call both sorts of problem "sickness.") Without sickness or the threat of sickness, the institution of clinical medicine would cease to exist. The general trend is familiar: I get sick, I go to the doctor. There are, of course, variations: I am concerned that I might be getting sick—perhaps after I notice that my skin has taken on a strange hue—or I am concerned that I might get sick in the future—perhaps I have a family history of hypertension—so I go to the doctor. Sickness, then, is the efficient cause of the clinical dyad.

But if sickness, viewed as an evil, is the precondition for the clinical dyad, then the eradication, prevention, or mitigation of sickness is its aim. That is to say, the purpose, or final cause, of the clinical dyad is to help the patient get rid of and/or stay free from sickness or the effects of sickness. It is around this task that the physician organizes all professional efforts.

Finally, it is through the utilization of scientific research and technological advancement that the physician carries out his or her task. The formal cause of the clinical dyad consists of its conceptual apparatus and its fund of technical procedures, as well as the formal relations of authority, knowledge, responsibility, and power that characterize clinical medicine as it is now practiced.

Under these relations and methodologies, the sickness—that all-important problem that was born out of the experience of patients—usually undergoes a curious transformation. This transformation is familiar to students of medical philosophy, but it is worth a review. "Sickness," as it occurs from the frame of reference of one who is sick, is a disruption. It is a state of existence where the individual is unable to carry on with his usual activities or is unable to derive the same level of satisfaction from life. Often, this disruption takes the form of physical pain or discomfort, such that the stream of consciousness is constantly disrupted by unpleasant or excruciating qualities, perceived to be of somatic origin. But other manifestations are common as well—dizziness, tingling sensations, weakness, loss of appetite, too great an appetite, uncomfortable sensations of cold or heat, fuzzy vision, buzzing in the ears, bowel irregularities, changes in appearance, fluttering in the chest, mood swings, sexual malfunction, or the feeling that one's uvula is gyrating. What all these qualities have in common is that, for individuals who think of themselves as sick, they are qualities experienced as problems. They are suffered. If they were perceived as acceptable aspects of experience, devoid of negative connotations, they would never be classified as symptoms of sickness.

Enter our physician. The patient seeks her help in eradicating his sickness. This process occurs in several stages. First, the patient tells about his suffering, describing his experiences in his own words.[3] He will describe how and when these experiences have occurred, and, perhaps upon questioning, will reveal whether he has had similar experiences in the past, and, if so, what was done about them. He may also elaborate on other related prior illnesses or conditions, medications, and allergies. This stage can be brief or extended, depending on factors such as the physician's schedule, the loquaciousness of the patient, and how severe or important the problem seems to be in the view of the patient or physician. Next comes an act of translation. The physician reads the tingling sensation in the elbow as a paresthesia, the fluttering in the chest as a palpitation, and the "cruddy" feeling as malaise. Third, there is a laying on of hands—often the most therapeutic aspect of the clinical encounter—when the physician examines the patient. These first three steps, classified by the physician as the history and physical exam (H&P) generally form the basis for a diagnosis, often provisional in nature, or a series of possible diagnoses—the "differential diagnosis." If the diagnosis derived from the H&P is felt to be uncertain (or "insecure," as physicians often say), further diagnostic tests are usually ordered, until the physician feels confident that she has the right diagnosis or has accumulated good reasons for no longer caring about a secure diagnosis. The final diagnosis is the physician's version of the "sickness."

The "sickness," then, as it is perceived by the physician, is something quite different from the "sickness" of the patient. For the patient it is suffering—pervasive, invasive, and subjective. For the physician, it is a challenge—isolatable and objective. Let us henceforth use the term *illness* when referring to "sickness" as it is perceived or conceived by our patient, and *disease* as it is viewed by the physician. The illness and the disease are never quite identical.

Recall that Royce defines the human self as a life lived according to a plan. It is important that we view the patient's illness within the framework of this notion of selfhood. The most devastating illnesses derive their notoriety from their impact on the patient's life plan. These illnesses are problematic because they prevent patients from pursuing their ideals. Even the patient who seems wholly uncommitted to any cause will generally be concerned to safeguard his or her own comfort and in this sense has an ideal, selfish and narrow though it be. The patient who lacks even this basic sort of life plan will be impervious to illness (though, of course, not to disease) and, therefore, comes only infrequently under the care of a physician.

Often, a patient's perception of suffered illness evolves with the unfolding clinical inquiry, emerging, supposedly under the tutelage of the physician, from the murky water of feelings into the clear sunlight of objectivity. When such a transformation occurs, the patient's illness takes on many of the characteristics of the disease, as understood by the physician. It is also the case—more often when physicians are good listeners—that the disease is modified by contact with the illness. That is, the physician is apt to revise estimation of the disease by interpreting it in light of the patient's suffering. Zaner summarizes the process:

> It seems perfectly obvious that what the healer observes is in almost all cases an embodied person who both experiences and interprets his own distress, illness, or damage and, in one way or another, does this both for himself and for the healer. Indeed, in continuous interaction with the healer, patients both experience and interpret themselves in this complex manner, and both patient and physician continuously respond to and interpret their respective shared interpretations. (1988, 173)

Nevertheless, the illness always has a qualitative dimension that exceeds the disease. It is out of this dimension that the whole enterprise of clinical medicine develops. Apart from the subjective experience of patients, modern theories of pathophysiology would be no more than useless meanderings. Talk about "disease" is useful only because diseases relate to illnesses. Moderately high levels of lipids in the blood, for instance, were of no interest and were not considered "disease" until the medical community correlated them with atherosclerosis, which is considered a disease because of its association with several effects that many people experience as unpleasant or otherwise undesirable (such as chest pain, hemiparalysis, and death). Apart from the relation to atherosclerosis, or to some other illness-causing factor, the investigation of moderate hyperlipidemia would be pointless. The priority of illness over disease is the central lesson of medical phenomenology, such as we see explored in the works of Zaner and Cassell, and it is the springboard of our discussion of loyalty in the clinical dyad.

We have specified that loyalty within the context of the clinical dyad will be devotion to the interests or ideals of the dyad conceived as a community. We have examined those interests and are now in a position to formulate them. The ideal of the clinical dyad is to utilize scientific knowledge and technological innovation in order to assist the patient by intervening in current illnesses and/or preventing future illnesses. Take note: We have defined the ideal of the clinical dyad in terms of a fight against illness, not against disease. Our physician, then, could be classified as the loyal physician, in one view at least, because she is devoted to the realization of this ideal and expresses this devotion through utilizing her special training and skills.[4]

Certain aspects of the clinical dyad distinguish it from other communities and will affect the way this ideal is served. First, there is an asymmetry of responsibility. It is the physician who incurs the most burdensome obligations. She is the one who is expected to conform to the most rigorous standards. If she strays from accepted practice, she may be sued, stripped of her license, or otherwise reprimanded. Second, there is an asymmetry of control. The patient is the one who initiates the clinical encounter. He is (or should be) the one who has the most control over fashioning the community ideal (that is, in defining the state of wellness or relief from suffering). The physician, on the other hand, is largely in control of diagnostic testing, final diagnosis and therapy. She also has the benefit of functioning in a familiar environment and is presumably in good health. She is bestowed, largely by virtue of these factors, with security, clearheadedness, and confidence to a degree that generally eludes the patient. Third, due to the aforementioned asymmetries, the ideal of the clinical dyad is a degenerate cause (in a way we will soon examine). Loyalty to the ideal of the clinical dyad, as we will see, lacks some of the characteristics of true loyalty. Fourth, the dyadic character of this community is morally dangerous and requires that the community be subject to the influence of mediating communities. I will not discuss the first two of these aspects now (the asymmetries of responsibility and control). But comment is due, I believe, on the third and fourth, that the clinical dyad is a degenerate cause and that it is morally dangerous.

It is not difficult to show that the patient's obligations to the clinical dyad amount to less than a genuine call to loyalty. Though it is reasonable that our patient should be obliged to cooperate in his care—otherwise the solicitation of our physician would be disingenuous—the ideal that this care aims to achieve is nothing other than a restoration or preservation of the patient's personal well-being, as defined by the patient himself. In other words, the ideal of the community, from the viewpoint of the patient, does not eclipse his own life. There would be, in fact, no dyad at all were it not for the patient and the peculiar needs he brings into the relationship. In this sense, the ideal of the clinical dyad, from the frame of reference of the patient, lacks the transpersonal quality upon which Royce insists—it is not a "cause" in the Roycean sense. For the same reason, it is not a cause for the physician. The loyalty of the physician to the ideal of the clinical dyad comes too close to what most would express as loyalty to an individual. But Royce has insisted that loyalty is never loyalty merely to a single human individual. In his account, true loyalty, when it exists in dyadic communities, is loyalty to a tie that binds the two members, a tie that transcends their respective personalities. But in the case of the clinical dyad, the ideal of the community is largely circumscribed within the boundaries of the patient's individual experience.

One may be tempted to counter on at least two points: (1) the ideal is never wholly fashioned by the patient—our physician contributes her own insights, derived from sources beyond herself, and these insights, in turn, influence the metamorphosis of the patient's conception of his illness; and (2) the process of healing or the promotion of health is part of a grander process that is unfolding throughout the world; it has implications that extend beyond both members of the dyad. Both these considerations are certainly true. But they bespeak the fact that the clinical dyad is itself a sort of individual, having many of the characteristics of a person, including a relationship with larger social groups. The dyad still lacks an important characteristic that even the relationship between lovers can claim—the genesis of a new, unique ideal, according to which each member of the community is more or less equally responsible for creating, nurturing, and developing something that far exceeds what the individual could envisage singly.[5]

The fourth aspect distinguishing the clinical dyad from other communities was its potential instability. Any dyadic community, according to Royce, that does not consciously appeal to a mediating community will be unstable. He expresses this instability in two laws:

> When two men, or two consolidated groups of men, are set at some such social task as observing each other, or playing a game together, or debating a question, or buying and selling, or borrowing and lending, or hunting for food, or even when they explicitly undertake the task of helping each other, then, at any one stage of this dual or bilateral activity, one of the two will indeed be either loving the other, or else not loving him. And when a new and interesting relation to a neighbor first comes in sight, love is quite as natural as antipathy. But as the two individuals pass from one stage to another of the activity in question, the natural contrast between the two men or groups tends to lead to some mutual interruption, of jostling, or to some other vexatious contrast of behavior. Each therefore tends, in some fashion, to surprise the other painfully, to snub his activities, and so to get in the other's way. We naturally do such things not because we are by nature either mainly selfish or primarily malicious or even greedy. We do all this merely because, if taken in pairs, we are, in each pair, two different and contrasting people or groups. Our whole self-consciousness, in fact, depends upon noting how different from our neighbors each of us is. But contrasts that strongly interest us can easily become unpleasant. . . . The second half of our law is easily stated. When mutual friction once arises between a pair of lovers or of rivals or of individuals otherwise in-

terestingly related, whether they be men or groups of men, *the friction tends to increase*, unless some other relation intervenes. . . . (WAR, 32–35)

These laws can be summarized: (1) dyadic relations engender conflict; (2) conflicts within dyadic relations tend to escalate.

The clinical dyad should, theoretically, be susceptible to these Roycean laws. I believe that it is. Insofar as it is conceived by the parties as exclusively a dyad—that is, insofar as both the physician and the patient recognize no higher ideal than the interests of the dyadic community—conflict is bound to emerge. This problem is evidenced by the failure of what I call the entrepreneurial model of the physician-patient relationship. Within the entrepreneurial relationship the physician is regarded as a businessman, enlisted by his customer, the patient, in order to provide needed services for a fee. The moral obligations engendered by this relationship are expressed in a version of contractualism.

The clinical dyad is conceived in the entrepreneurial model at the first level of morality. Both the physician and the patient are viewed as essentially selfish. The major concern of the physician is making a profit. The major concern of the patient is his health. The physician sees to it that the patient's health is promoted, but only because this activity is profitable. The patient sees to it that the physician is paid, but only because he would otherwise be unable to enlist future services. There may sometimes be affection or mutual concern between physician and patient. However, such attitudes are always only a kind of excess baggage, never an ideal, never an integral part of the business relationship. So conceived, the clinical dyad is not a community—it contains no central mutually held ideal.[6]

Because of this lack of an ideal, distrust is likely to develop within the dyadic relationship. Distrust, of course, engenders conflict. Our physician comes to resent certain patients whom she perceives as "abusing the system"—usually those who make a lot of work for her, without substantially contributing to her remuneration. This class of patients often includes, among others, government-sponsored patients (for instance, those who pay through Medicare or Medicaid), uninsured patients who do not pay, uncooperative patients (especially those with self-inflicted illness or foul dispositions), and managed-care patients who show up when or where the physician thinks they should not. Our patient, especially if he fits into one of the above categories, often perceives that the physician is motivated by something other than the patient's best interests (a perception that should generate neither surprise nor condemnation from those who uphold the entrepreneurial model; yet somehow it usually does). The patient begins to wonder if his physician should be ordering more (or fewer) X rays or blood tests. If he has a viral illness, the patient may have a preconceived notion that he needs antibiotics, and rather than trusting the physician's assessment that he does not, may suspect that her recommendations represent ulterior concerns. If the physician recommends surgery, the patient is likely to wonder if this procedure is more necessary for the proverbial Mercedes payment than it is for health. And patients of all sorts will tend to be upset that their physicians are not willing to spend more time with them, while also lamenting how long they waited while their physician was tending to the previous patient. In a manner akin to the escalation described by Royce, the dyadic relation between physician and patient tends to develop friction.

Clearly, this failure of the entrepreneurial model is the fate of any version of the physician-patient relation that insists on conceiving the relation in merely dyadic terms. Our first model of the clinical dyad differed from the entrepreneurial model in that both physician and patient were primarily concerned to promote the health of the patient. But even the more ideal dyadic relationship is doomed if we do not invoke a mediating community. Two major reasons for this prognosis emerge. First, the two parties will never agree about how best to promote health (the logistical problem) unless they agree on what scientific theories and technologies are authoritative. This involves an appeal to several mediating communities.[7] For instance, recall our patient wanting antibiotics for a viral illness. He does not believe the physician when she tells him they are not helpful for his condition. Now suppose patient and physician have forged the ideal kind of dyadic clinical relation that we outlined earlier. The patient is confident that the physician is dedicated to promoting his health. Nevertheless, he questions the wisdom of her judgment. In this case, conflict will, once again, arise. This conflict can be resolved only if both parties agree about the authority of some higher community. The physician can explain the scientific rationale for antibiotic therapy. Perhaps she will cite specific studies or provide the patient with educational pamphlets prepared by a scientific organization such as the CDC (Centers for Disease Control). These measures should bring about agreement if both parties acknowledge the authority of the community of scientific researchers. The tension engendered by the dyadic relation will have been mediated. But for a second reason we will soon find that other difficulties will arise within the physician-patient relation that require appeals to mediating communities beyond the research community in authority.

The second reason behind the dismal prognosis for the dyadic relationship in question is that our physician is not a unidimensional altruist, dedicated entirely to the needs of her patients. Her involvement in the clinical dyad always includes a concern for remuneration, reflecting her devotion to other ideals, such as the financial security of her family. In other words, the loyal physician will always have causes other than the ideal of the clinical dyad. Insofar as she is motivated by profit, the entrepreneurial model will accurately reflect her posture. Our critique of this model can never be that it misses reality entirely, only that it is too narrow. To insure that the entrepreneurial concerns of the physician and the selfishness of the patient do not lead to the victimization of the other party, there must be an appeal to a third party.[8] The solution, then, to the ailments of the clinical dyad, is in mediation. This, of course, is exactly what Royce suggests.

MEDIATING THE PHYSICIAN-PATIENT RELATION

Consider the plight of Dr. Wascher. She is an orthopedist who is called to the ER to see Mr. Storaasli. Mr. Storaasli has a bimaleolar fracture of his ankle. It is an unstable fracture and must be treated operatively if Mr. Storaasli is to have any hope of recovering the strength in his ankle. Dr. Wascher examines him and informs him that surgery is absolutely mandatory in situations such as his. Mr. Storaasli understands but is frightened by the idea of having surgery. His fear of surgery dates back to an episode of *Dr. Kildare* he saw during his childhood. Because of this fear, Mr. Storaasli declines Dr. Wascher's recommendation. He requests, instead, that Dr. Wascher caste his extremity, provide him with crutches and analgesics, and recommend the best possible nonoperative treatment. Dr. Wascher is not inclined to go along with this suggestion. To be party to such a plan would be, in Dr. Wascher's opinion, tantamount to engaging in malpractice. Dr. Wascher and Mr. Storaasli argue back and forth. Though both agree that the purpose of their association is to alleviate or ameliorate Mr. Storaasli's suffering, they cannot come to terms on how this should be accomplished. Their disagreement seems irresoluble.

Royce's solution to the problem of the instability of dyadic relations, and the conflicts they engender, is to convert traditionally dyadic relations into polyadic ones by enlisting mediators. With the goal of shedding light on how this could work in the case of the clinical dyad, we will backtrack temporarily to the discussion of general triadic relations.

Recall that the principal, interpreter, and interpretant are all signs. What sorts of signs may serve as the elements in an interpretive process? On the one hand, any creative process of interpretation must include a sign that is a thought-sign, or a complex of thought-signs, such as a person or group. On the other hand, any sort of thing—a physical object, a physical process, a thought, a person, a group of persons—may serve as one of the elements of the triad. Thus, the triad of principal-interpreter-interpretant may take on a huge variety of possible structures. It could be composed of a physical object, a person, and a group—as when a lecturer in chemistry explains the structure of his notebook to a group of students. It could be composed of three groups—as when the United Nations counsels one nation on behalf of another. It could be composed of three thoughts—as when a sensation is correlated with the thought of some cause by the mediating idea of a pain-producing mechanism. The permutations are numerous.

What about structural relations between the elements of a triad? Once again, we find several possibilities. Each sign may be relatively independent of the others—as in the example of the chemistry professor. On the other hand, the principal and/or the interpretant could be elements of the mediator—as in the example of the United Nations—or the mediator might be an element of what it mediates—as when a mother discusses her country with family members.

Often a single interpretive event may be accurately represented in several different ways. Of supreme importance is the way we choose to interpret the interaction between human selves. When Gerta interacts with Mike, does she interpret Mike's thoughts, or only her own thoughts about Mike? Royce holds that none of us has firsthand experience of the thoughts of others, and thus, none of us has ever directly verified the presence of other thinkers in our universe (PC 313, 324).[9] Nevertheless, our entire way of life is dependent on the fact that we believe in the existence of others like ourselves. It is essential that, on some level, Gerta is able to view herself as interpreting Mike's thoughts and not just her own. This is an act of empathy; its importance may be traced back to early human development.

The human infant begins to conceive of itself as a self only after imitating (the will of) a model. The process of imitation, quite obviously, requires empathy—the infant must view the model as a being with an inner life and then interpret that life in an act of imitation. This perceptiveness of infants is the germ of the moral insight. All of us, as we grow, need to view ourselves as members of a community, and to conceive of community we must, once again, conceive of interpersonal communication—we must be willing to assert that we and others are able, however imperfectly, to interpret the thoughts of others. The importance of this assertion—this faith in the potential for community life—is manifest even in the life of the objective sciences.

The dependence of science on the notion of a community of interpreters is manifest on several levels. Let us begin by looking at the process of theorization.[10] The theorist begins by observing an event or, more likely, a large number of similar events. Suppose, for instance, that a man becomes intrigued with balloons. He notices that every balloon has a flaccid area near the knot, and he wonders if this familiar phenomenon can be described in terms of a law. He hypothesizes that it is a manifestation of a general law that the wall tension of any hollow distensible object is related to the pressure within the object and the radii of curvature of the object—$T = P/(1/Ra + 1/Rb)$.[11] He may devise a method of tentatively verifying this hypothesis. Eventually, if all goes well, he will present it to other investigators.

I would like to comment on two aspects of this brief scenario. First, the theorist's conceptualization of the event to be explained is itself an interpretation of the inner life of others. He presupposes that his experience of an asymmetry in wall tension has been duplicated in the experience of countless others and recurs whenever people encounter balloons. In other words, his hypothesis, insofar as it is a scientific hypothesis, is an interpretation of an aspect of the collective life of a large group of persons. One does not make a scientific hypothesis to explain why pink elephants float across bedroom ceilings—such an event is not part of humanity's collective experience. Instead, one hypothesizes about why persons who have imbibed more than a fifth of whiskey frequently hallucinate—because a relation between intoxication and such experiences is (or is interpreted to be) an aspect of our collective experience. Our theorist, then, is part of a triad in which: (1) the principal is all of humanity; (2) the interpreter is the theorist; and (3) the interpretant can be designated as the hypothesis, or, in a broader view, the scientific community to whom the hypothesis is addressed.[12] Recall that each interpretant is, or potentially is, a principal. This consideration leads us to the next point.

The hypothesis (or the hypothesizer) will be the principal in acts of interpretation that antedate its acceptance within the scientific community. Royce describes the process:

> The scientific community consists, at the least, of the original discoverer, of his interpreter, and of the critical worker who tests or controls the discoverer's observations by means of new experiences devised for that purpose. (PC 331)

Once again, the life of science is expressed in terms of a community of interpretation.[13]

The interpreter in scientific communities, as described by Royce, is one who explains, and derives the consequences from, the hypotheses generated by theorists, in order that others may work to verify it. There are, accordingly, three functional roles within the scientific community: (1) theorist (the principal); (2) interpreter; and (3) researcher (the interpretant). It is possible, of course, for one individual to play all three roles at different times. But no researcher, not even our balloon theorist, is ever credited with singlehandedly proving his own theory. After he has generated a hypothesis, gone on to interpret it himself in terms of an experimental design, and then carried out his experiment, he has only begun the process. He now suggests to other interpreters how they should approach his theory. He suggests to other researchers what they might do to verify it and what results he has preliminarily obtained. This is all that one person can do. From here on there is a mandatory social review of his project. The necessity of such a review is expressed in Minot's thesis:

In that lecture "On the Method of Science" Professor Minot carefully expounded, and very extensively illustrated, the thesis that, while natural science is dependent upon the experiences of individuals for every one of its advances in the knowledge of the facts of nature, no experience of any individual man can count as a scientific discovery until it has been sufficiently confirmed by other and by independent observers. (PC, 322)

Royce's model of the scientific community is important to our discussion of the clinical dyad for two reasons. First, the clinical dyad, as we have intimated, is informed by the scientific community. We will say more about this soon. Second, the model of the scientific community is closely analogous to the model of the greater medical community, which I now wish to offer as a theoretical and practical basis for mediating the clinical dyad.

I will use, interchangeably, two names—*the greater medical community* and *the concerned public*—to designate a community that is defined as the community of all persons who are interested in utilizing and/or advancing the knowledge, customs, and methods that have emerged during the history of clinical medicine, with the aim of furthering the health and alleviating or mitigating the suffering of human beings. I will not offer a precise definition of what I mean by "suffering" or "health." It is important that both be studied at greater length than I can afford here, and such an effort is probably not much aided by a definition.

Two points, however, deserve emphasis. First, suffering and health, while intimately related, are not reciprocals. Cassell has done much to advance our understanding of suffering. His dictum, "The only way to learn whether suffering is present is to ask the sufferer," should be heeded (Cassell 1991, 44). The same is not true of health. One can be ignorant of one's unhealth. Such a person can be unhealthy (for instance, she may have ovarian cancer) even though she is not suffering. Further, not all suffering is related to ill health. I may suffer because my tax return is being audited or because my carburetor malfunctions, but these complaints are not related to my health and are not the concern of medicine. Nevertheless, health is closely related to suffering, since, as we have observed, we regard only those conditions that eventuate in human suffering as embodiments of ill health. This leads to the second point of emphasis. Even though suffering is not the exclusive province of medicine, physical suffering, rather than health, is medicine's originative concern. If our pursuit of the good life were not subject to the ravages of physical suffering and death, the practice of medicine would never have evolved, and the concept of health would be pointless.

The importance of the greater medical community, or concerned public, derives from the fact that both the patient and the physician are members. It deserves the loyalty of both. It has, we will find, immediate authority over the conflicts arising between the physician and patient. But the greater medical community includes more than just doctors and patients. It includes a multiplicity of subgroups. These include: (1) the clinical community, comprised of physicians, nurses, PAs, EMTs, paramedics, X-ray and respiratory technicians, pharmacists, and other persons involved directly in patient care, (2) the research community, comprised of doctors, nurses and other scientists who are devoted to research in the medical sciences; (3) several ancillary communities (for instance, those including health-policy makers, health-care administrators, lawyers specializing in medicolegal affairs, and lab technicians) having specific nonclinical, nonresearch roles that serve the ideal of the greater medical community, and (4) the lay public, defined as the group of patients or prospective patients who do not belong to clinical, research or ancillary communities.

The reader is cautioned about three possible confusions. First, the "concerned public" should not be confused with what I will call the "general public." Though the membership of each of these groups is essentially the same—virtually everyone in the state, province, or country—the former community is circumscribed by a narrower range of concerns. The concerned public is the general public insofar as it is devoted to the ideal of quality health care (which is why it can also be called the greater medical community). It is possible for the goals of the concerned public to conflict with the overarching goals of the general public. Second, neither the general public nor the concerned public should be confused with the lay public. This latter group does not include those who work in the provision of health care; the first two do. Third, the "greater medical community" should not be confused with the various groups that have, from time to time, been dubbed "medical community." Such groups—perhaps we should call them versions of the "plain old medical community"—are composed of various combinations of people who earn a living through the health care industry. If I speak of the "medical community" alone, I will be referring to the community composed of both clinicians and researchers. But when I speak of the "greater medical community" I refer to all the groups that we enumerated when we defined this community. The reader should not forget that the greater medical community and the concerned public are identical.

It is evident that talk of the physician-patient relation as the molecule of the medical establishment is overly restrictive. Satisfactory clinical outcomes can be achieved without physicians (as, for instance, when a nurse practitioner does a well-baby check and treats an infant for a monilial diaper rash, or when a pharmacist aids someone in the proper selection of an over-the-counter medication). There are many varieties of clinical encounter. We are concerned in this study with the professional life of physicians, and so we will not treat these other professions in detail. But it is important to understand that the physician is not the indispensable common denominator of clinical medicine. That role belongs to the patient alone.

Let us return to the clinical relation between patient and physician. In our original case described at the outset of this chapter, the patient has come to the physician because he is concerned about an illness. In our initial discussion, we described this encounter as an exchange of services for money, so that the knowledge, skills, and technology that the patient desires to use are conceived as the property of the physician, which she will dispense. A more natural description is suggested by our discussion of communities of interpretation. Rather than a possessor of truth, skills, and technology, we can conceive the physician as an interpreter. It is from the concepts and tools of medical science that the patient hopes to benefit; the office of the physician is to make these things available to her patient by correlating them with his symptoms and signs.

The physician—as an agent of the scientific community—interprets the patient's illness to the patient. Ultimately, then, patients are the principals and the interpretants. The patient experiences a problem—he feels ill. This experience is the principal sign from which the continuum of interpretations that constitute the clinical endeavor follow. He interprets his problem to be something warranting medical attention. He visits his physician and tells her about his problem (which is another act of interpretation). The physician then performs two acts of interpretation at once. She reinterprets his story, using the language of medicine, while interpreting medical science to him by explaining relevant pathophysiology and interventions. He then decides how he will utilize the physician's recommendations (he interprets them to himself), and he lives with the results. He is the final interpretant. The story of medicine begins and ends with those who get sick.

The physician, in the above account, is a two-way mediator, facilitating a dialogue between the patient and the medical community. She mediates in two directions. First, she interprets the knowledge of the research community to the patient. This process is familiar. The role of the physician here is to correlate the truths, the techniques, and the technology of medical science with the illness of the patient. This activity is perfectly analogous to the acts of "correlation" that Royce and Minot describe as the role of interpreters within any scientific community (PC, 331). Thus, the greater medical community—including researchers, clinicians, and patients—is an analogue of Minot's community of research. Interestingly, it also includes the research community as one of its members.

But the clinician directs her interpretations otherwise than just toward the patient. She also interprets the patient to the research community. We have noted that it is the business of the researcher to interpret humanity's collective experience. In our original example of the balloon theorist (the law of Laplace), the researcher attempted to explain the common experience of areas of flaccidity near the knots on balloons. Medical researchers, analogously, try to explain common forms of physical suffering. They are dependent upon clinicians for the data constituting their subject matter. And these data are compiled through the interpretation, by clinicians, of their patients' suffering.

For instance, in 1975 clinicians in Lyme, Connecticut, began seeing clusters of children who complained of joint pain. Most had inflammatory arthropathy. The clinicians relayed this information to researchers, who named the malady "Lyme arthritis." With the cooperation of clinicians and their patients, researchers gathered more data. They learned that Lyme arthritis was no mere childhood disease. It affected people of all ages. Clinicians soon correlated the arthritis with prodromal symptoms—a red rash that migrated out from the site of a tick bite, and a mild flu-like illness that followed shortly thereafter. They also noted that many persons with the characteristic prodrome went on to develop carditis or neurological derangements. This information was passed on to researchers, who soon traced the illness to deer ticks. Seven years after the first children presented with sore joints in Connecticut, the etiologic agent of Lyme Disease was discovered—a spirochete, *Borrelia burgdorferi*.

None of this would have occurred if the kids had not complained about their joints, if their parents had not thought these complaints warranted medical attention, and if the physicians had not reported the events to researchers. There can be no research without field work. In medicine, the field work is done by clinicians and patients. Without their participation, there would be nothing to research. This truth may occasionally be obscured by the fact that many researchers are themselves clinicians. But recall Minot. None of these clinician-researchers can singlehandedly prove their own theories. We should add that none of them can singlehandedly isolate the problems that warrant research.

We have indicated that both the physician and the patient will have a dual citizenship. The patient is a member of the lay public and also of the greater medical community. The physician is a member of the clinical community and also the greater medical community. These affiliations are attended by obligations.

The physician is expected to be loyal to the clinical community. Like any community, the clinical community is not an organization but consists of the actual union of its members, through the recognition of common ideals, in the manner we have previously described. Nevertheless, there are organizations that are founded more or less centrally on the notion of a clinical community. The American Medical Association, the American College of Emergency Physicians, and local medical societies are examples. The smaller regional and specialty societies may be viewed, for our present purposes, as suborganizations that correlate with subcommunities within the clinical community. Sir William Osler lectured about the virtues of the medical society in 1903. His account bears repetition. In it we find the mission of the clinical community.

To quote Osler:

> The first, and in some respects the most important, function [of the medical society] is that mentioned by the wise founders of your parent society—to lay a foundation for that unity and friendship which is essential to the dignity and usefulness of the profession. (Osler 1932, 335)

The office of unity and friendship belongs within all real communities. It is one of the ways that we augment and reinfuse the fragile loyalties of our members.

The other function of the medical society, according to Osler, is the maintenance of professional competence:

> The well-conducted medical society should represent a clearing house, in which every physician of the district would receive his intellectual rating, and in which he could find out his professional assets and liabilities. (337)

Competence, according to Jonsen, was the trademark virtue of Osler and his contemporary Cabot. Osler recommends that medical societies can be used as forums for the presentation of case histories and anatomy specimens and also as sites for medical libraries.

Both of these functions of medical societies point toward a greater mission—service to the concerned public. Neither the unity of clinicians nor their competence would be meaningful apart from a devotion to the treatment and prevention of illness, which is the ideal of the concerned public and the overarching purpose of all its member communities.

Thus, our paradigmatic physician, through her loyalty to the clinical community, takes on an obligation to the concerned public or greater medical community. What this obligation involves is determined largely by the operative form of the medical tradition and how she interprets it. We have indicated that this tradition is in need of modification—that will be the topic of the next chapter.

Our patient is also called to be loyal to the concerned public. Some may find this claim confusing. Nevertheless, the basis of the patient's obligation is straightforward. Two primary considerations imply it. First, the concerned public is the essential cause of the whole endeavor of clinical medicine—apart from this group, and its collective experience, no medical community could exist; in fact, without it the individual patient would be without a means of expressing the discomfort of his illness. This point warrants restatement. Clinical medicine is a science. Science, as we have pointed out twice in detail, is possible only in the context of shared experience. If the individual who suffers from physical discomfort has no fellow sufferers, there is no basis for a scientific approach to his ailment. He will be entirely alone with his illness, deprived of support or hope.

The second source of the patient's obligation to the greater medical community derives from his membership in this community. Fairness demands that, if the patient expects he will receive expedient and competent attention within the medical complex, he must be a part of a public effort to maintain it. The patient's obligation to the concerned public is, in fact, a function of his obligation to the general public of which he is a citizen (say, his country and his state or province). The ideal of the concerned public or greater medical community has arisen out of the will of the general public, and it demands the loyalty of the general public, just as the concerned public, in turn, loyally serves the general public. More obligations inhere within the domain of the general public than just a commitment to the greater medical community. This situation is paradigmatic of one kind of moral relation between groups. Both communities are composed of the same persons but serve different functions. They should be mutually loyal—the subordinate community (the concerned public or greater medical community) should be loyal because of its subordination; the principal community (the general public) shoould be loyal because of its originative will.

The reader may have noted that I have not claimed that the patient ought to be loyal to the lay public. That claim is withheld purposefully. I use the term "lay public" to designate all actual or potential patients who are not health care workers.[14] The lay public is not a community. Because it is not a community, it does not command loyalty. It is a population of persons who are prone to physical suffering. Since one may suffer alone, without being aware or concerned about the suffering of others, there is nothing about this group committing its members to a common memory or expectation. Insofar as they have such memories or expectations, related to a common desire for health and the avoidance of physical suffering, they are members of the concerned public. As members of the lay public they need have only their individual concerns.

Nevertheless, the lay public has its importance. As Zaner and Cassell remind us, the experience of individuals includes suffering. Corresponding with the uniqueness of individuals is the uniqueness of their suffering. Though it would be impossible for them to express their distress outside the context of a community, with a common language and a common experience of similar sufferings, it is nevertheless their unique instances of suffering that call for resolution in particular clinical encounters. Jonsen tells us that "the new medicine" sees patients increasingly as members of a class (1990, 30). Nevertheless, keeping their individuality in mind is important. Even given that the true meaning of personhood is loyalty to a community, patients will have their own unique blends of loyalties. They will be loyal to other causes besides the ideal of the concerned public. And they will serve this variety of causes, each in his or her own way.

Given these considerations, preserving the individuality of patients becomes a paramount concern of the greater medical community. It may seem paradoxical, but the larger group—the greater medical community—which commands the loyalty of the individual, is itself committed, above all else, to maintaining and cultivating the dignity and self-actualization of the individual. This is the paradox of self-realization revisited. Only with an ethics of loyalty can the inevitable tension between the demands of such a community and the needs of the individual be resolved. Only through loyalty can the physician serve members of the lay public without being thwarted by self-interest or impersonalism.

Earlier we noted that dyadic relations, such as the physician-patient relation we originally portrayed, are unstable, that the parties in the relation will be prone to escalating conflict. We noted that this tendency is partially counteracted by an internal mechanism for resolving conflict within the clinical dyad. In distinction to many other sorts of dyadic relationship, both parties of the clinical dyad will be primarily committed to a single goal—alleviating the suffering of the patient. But we now see that this commitment is based on more than a contractual relation between the two parties. It is based on mutual loyalty to the greater medical community. Our recognition of this loyalty corresponds to our discovery of the basis by which conflicts, unresolvable by mere reference to the opinions or desires of the patient, can be mediated.

We asked if there were parties that could mediate conflicts within the clinical dyad. Our answer is now at hand. There are three important mediators. First, there is the clinical community. Because the physician is loyal to this community, he may look to it for guidance when he is confronted by the patient. Occasionally, this will be as far as he has to look. Take the case of Dr. Baize. She wants to treat Mr. Threecoat's migraine headache with 50 milligrams of IM Thorazine, but Mr. Threecoat opposes this strategy because he doesn't want to take a heavily sedating medication. If Dr. Baize consults with the local neurologist or ED physician, she is apt to learn that intravenous Reglan is being used for similar headaches and is at least as effective as IM Thorazine, but far less sedating. The conflict is resolved by an appeal to the clinical community.

A second mediating community is the research community. Suppose Dr. Anderson wants to get a CBC and blood cultures on the eighteen-month-old he is seeing because of fever. These tests are standard in the emergency department where he works. But his patient's mother doesn't want the child to undergo the pain experienced when blood is drawn. If Dr. Anderson has an adequate database on hand, and stops to consult it, he will find recent data showing that CBCs and blood cultures contribute virtually nothing to the management of most nontoxic 18-month-olds with fever. His conflict is resolved by an appeal to the research community.

Unfortunately, appealing to these communities will not always provide answers. Recall Dr. Wascher's conflict with Mr. Storaasli. It cannot be resolved by appealing to the medical or to the research community. If Dr. Wascher appeals to the clinical community, she will be told that fractures of the sort experienced by Mr. Storaasli have to be opened, reduced, and internally fixated. The same guidance will come from the research community. Neither of these mediators has a well-developed system for dealing with Mr. Storaasli's unique manner of suffering, his dread of surgery.[15] Their standards are framed from the viewpoint of the biological sciences, which have not, as yet, collectively recognized a broad humanitarian foundation for their knowledge, such as the one proposed by Royce and Peirce. Cassell's words get to the root of Dr. Wascher's problem:

> From the scientific perspective . . . whether the man with a broken leg is in pain or the woman who has lost her hair from chemotherapy is suffering are questions which, not being open to empirical verification, can *never* be answered with certainty. If the question of whether someone is suffering is not open to scientific knowledge, then the relief of suffering—medicine's fundamental purpose—cannot be achieved by purely scientific medicine. (Cassell 1991, 176)

Insofar as the research or clinical communities do have a protocol for dealing with individual concerns such as Mr. Storaasli's, it is because they have already made an appeal to a higher community—the greater medical community. This appeal may have been based on a recognition that the deeper fundamental nature of science is constituted by its appeal to the inner experience of individuals. All the better if this is the case. More likely, at least in the current situation, such appeals are based on prudence.

Dr. Wascher must consult the greater medical community—the third mediating community. This community is an ideal mediator, we have remarked, because both patient and physician are called to loyalty to it. Three possible options are open to Dr. Wascher: (1) she could refuse to treat Mr. Storaasli in any but the accepted manner; (2) she could operate on Mr. Storaasli without consent (never mind, for now, that this would be illegal); or (3) she could institute temporizing therapy that Mr. Storaasli finds acceptable, while helping him to deal with his irrational fear of surgery. The first option is typical of those who view their mission in terms of a straightforward contractualist rule: The physician offers cutting-edge medical therapy, of proven efficacy, in her area of specialization. She is obliged to offer this therapy to the patient, who is obliged either to accept or reject it. This option, however, would not be approved by the greater medical community. Recall that the greater medical community is defined by the commitment to utilize and/or advance the knowledge, customs, and methods of clinical medicine, with the aim of furthering the health and alleviating or mitigating the suffering of human beings. The first option fails because it is not an efficient way of promoting health or mitigating suffering. It relieves both physician and patient too easily from the responsibility of searching for other ways of achieving this end, when the "standard" or "consensus" approach is not acceptable.

What about the second option? To operate on Mr. Storaasli without consent would be an act of brash paternalism. It could be justified by the consideration that Mr. Storaasli's reservations about surgery are not reasonable. Further, he would almost surely have a good outcome and, in the long run, would be healthier and suffer less than if surgery were not undertaken. However, two considerations (apart from its illegality) prohibit this move. First, the goal of alleviating Mr. Storaasli's suffering would not be served as well by this action as by the third option, pursuing temporizing therapy. By operating on Mr. Storaasli without consent, Dr. Wascher would undermine his trust in the medical establishment and consequently prejudice him against further therapeutic actions, should he become ill in the future. Further, the experience of being sedated and treated against his will could also lead to greater psychological distress for Mr. Storaasli. His suffering might even be increased by this action. Second, even supposing that Mr. Storaasli's suffering would be more effectively ameliorated by the second option than the third (perhaps because the delays inherent in the third option would lead to significantly more pain), this would still not be acceptable from the standpoint of the greater medical community. Why? Because the greater medical community—like all communities—must subordinate its ideals to the highest ideal, loyalty to loyalty. To operate on Mr. Storaasli against his will would be to violate his prerogative to serve his causes in the manner he chooses. It is unlikely that the spirit of loyalty, founded as it is on the decisions of individuals, could be cultivated by sanctioning the disregard of personal choice in this manner. Cassell is right to identify the proximal task of medicine as the relief (and we should add prevention) of suffering. But we must be cognizant of the requirement that this goal be served in the context of loyalty to loyalty.

It is the third option, then, that would be sanctioned by an appeal to higher communities. Once again, we observe how devotion to increasingly higher levels of community brings us ever closer to an appreciation for the sanctity of individual choices. Dr. Wascher could enlist the aid of psychologists, and possibly other family members, to help Mr. Storaasli deal with his fear of surgery. But to bring it off, Dr. Wascher will need to be loyal, not just to some rigid clinical standard but to her clinical relationship with Mr. Storaasli, to the greater medical community, and to loyalty itself.

To appeal to the greater medical community is to appeal to the moral tradition in medicine. My claim that this tradition is the property of the greater medical community may warrant more discussion than I have afforded it thus far. Recall that patients will point to this tradition when they are unsatisfied with the behavior of doctors. Patients' perception of the morality of medicine suggests that this tradition does not belong to medical professionals alone. A fuller justification of this claim lies in the consideration that medicine, even viewed from the perspective of medical professionals, is not the sort of activity that internally generates and maintains its own standards (as, for instance, some persons would say baseball does). It is through and through an enterprise defined by its relation with the greater community, and its tradition is generated by this relation. Ultimately, it is through the greater medical community and its tradition that the clinical dyad ought to be mediated. These considerations will be developed in the next chapter. However, let us first complete our discussion of the physician-patient relation by examining (1) how it embodies the three species of loyalty that Royce finds in families, and (2) how the notion of professional ethics would be altered under the conceptual scheme we have advocated for the physician-patient relation.

THREE SPECIES OF LOYALTY

We remarked in the chapter 3 that Royce identifies three distinct forms of loyalty that function within families, each with its correlative emphasis on one of the leading ideas of ethics. The relation between siblings was thought to center around the notion of autonomy; spouses were called to accentuate the notion of goodness; and within the parent-child relation, duty was emphasized. Once again, none of these relations is based solely on its correlative leading idea, and each of these species of loyalty is genuine only insofar as the related parties bring themselves willingly under the mediating influence of higher communities. Nevertheless, employing the aforementioned familial distinctions to call attention to the contextual nature of loyalty was helpful and may be relevant to our current enterprise as well.

Our notion of the physician-patient relation might be enriched if we note that each of the three familial species of loyalty must be at work within this relation if it is to manifest the integrity that we hope for. Physicians and patients must, first of all, bear quasi-sibling loyalties insofar as both physician and patient are called to respect the freedom of the other. The importance of respecting the autonomy of patients is an insight that has profoundly influenced contemporary medical ethics. We have underscored this insight by our discussion of the nature of illness: Each illness originates, we recall, from a disruption of the patient's life plan and therefore is contained only when this disruption is ameliorated. The goals of the clinical encounter, then, cannot be realized if clinical decision making is not directed by the autonomous choices of patients. On the other side of the coin, patients need to recognize the autonomy of physicians, not merely by allowing them to synthesize and utilize medicine's various resources in the way that each, in his or her uniqueness, can best serve the patient, but also by respecting the other loyalties of physicians. Among other things, this would entail that patients not expect their doctors to be on call twenty-four hours a day, seven days a week. From the perspective of their quasi-sibling loyalties, physicians and patients are able to see the grain of truth contained within the entrepreneurial model—that both patient and physician bring their own unique perspectives and life plans into the clinical encounter—and each must retain some freedom to interpret this encounter within the context of his or her broader outlook while safeguarding the other's freedom.

The quasi-spousal (or quasi-friendship) loyalty between physician and patient is founded on their common conception that clinical medicine is an aspect of the good life. This conception is apt to be based not merely on a common recognition of the value of health and the efficacy of modern medicine in preserving or restoring it, but also on the mutually perceived warmth and friendliness that characterize their association. Quasi-spousal loyalty is perhaps the most neglected aspect of standard treatments of the clinical encounter. For some reason, both organized medicine and bioethics have failed to celebrate the concrete goodness manifested by the fellowship between clinicians and patients. Apart from the loyal cultivation of such fellowship, I, personally, would find no joy in the practice of medicine.

A third kind of loyalty—that between parent and child—is manifested by an emphasis on complementary, but asymmetrical duties. The ethics of competence—with its emphasis on the physician's duty to stay current with medical knowledge—and various legalistic forms of ethics—which emphasize the duty to respect this or that right of the patient or to follow one principle or another—have already drawn attention to the serious responsibilities of physicians.[16] Less has been said about the duties of patients, but, as we have already indicated, these exist too. In addition to the duty to support the greater medical community in tangible ways (e.g., by supporting cancer research or by contributing to the construction of a community hospital), patients also have a duty to comply with a physician's advice, as long as that advice is given within the context of a genuine clinical relationship, is acceptable to the patient, and is consistent with the ideals of the greater medical community.

Within bioethics circles, the question of which of the aforementioned species of loyalty is most central to the physician-patient relation (sibling, spousal, or parent-child) underscores the conflict between an ethics of "autonomy" and an ethics of "beneficence." The "autonomy" school tends to view clinical relations in quasi-sibling terms (with an emphasis generally on respecting the autonomy of patients), the "beneficence" school in quasi-parent-child terms (thus the applied term *paternalism*). I submit that both parties miss the mark by exaggerating unidimensional perspectives. To wit, the asymmetry of function, power, and knowledge within the clinical relation limits the degree to which it can be considered a quasi-sibling relation, and the patient's (or patient representative's) mature standing within the greater medical community is not consistent with the parent-child model. We will have a great deal more to say about autonomy and beneficence in the next chapter.

As an aside, I think it would be worthwhile to investigate and characterize the interplay among these three species of loyalty as they function in the greater medical community outside the physician-patient relationship. Does the relationship between physician and nurse require a quasi-spousal loyalty, emphasizing the concrete good of their unity and cooperation? How about the relation between patient and patient—is it analogous to sibling relations, where the autonomy of each, in selecting modes of health care and being largely responsible for maintaining one's own health, ought to be emphasized? These are questions that will have to wait; but they deserve our attention.[17]

ON THE NOTION OF PROFESSIONAL ETHICS

Michael Hodges (1981) has suggested that we differentiate between two models of professional ethics. He calls one of these the activity model. It is premised by a claim about what it is to be a professional:

A professional is one who internalizes the standards of excellence of the activity that he engages in. In a sense he becomes the activity. His private motivation is identical with the standards of excellence that govern the activity.

Professional ethics, in this model, is the business of examining the nature of a professional activity and formulating the standards that are implicit in it. The values informing such a professional ethics are largely

what MacIntyre calls "goods internal to a practice." They have two defining characteristics: (1) they can be articulated only in terms of the specialized vocabulary of the activity; and (2) they can be fully recognized
and appreciated only by those who are experienced in the activity (AV
188–189). The purveyors of the activity model will generally recognize
the existence of some external good or goods that provide a basis for the
social importance of their profession. The internal standards are fashioned
with these external goods in mind, but they are, nonetheless, internal
standards, begetting internal goods.

Hodges calls the other model the contract model. Here, the standards
which comprise professional ethics are viewed as particular instances of a
general standard that applies to us all—the obligation to honor contracts.
Hodges elaborates:

> The general approach seems to be this. A profession is a social
> role to which a number of rights, duties and obligations attach.
> That is, it can be seen roughly as a sort of generalized "job de-
> scription." If, for example, the university defines the duties of a
> professor of philosophy as consisting in teaching 12 hours of
> classes, serving on 5 committees, publishing regularly and having
> office hours for 3 hours each week then, when I sign a contract
> with the university, I agree explicitly to take on those obligations
> in return for certain benefits that the university provides. It is im-
> portant to notice here that professional obligations and rights are
> in the first instance properties of certain social roles and only sec-
> ondarily properties of individuals who come to fill those roles.

He goes on to note that the social contract may be implicit or explicit.

The business of formulating a professional ethics, on the contract
model, consists of evaluating and balancing two concerns. First, we need
to determine which inducements will be offered to professionals. These
inducements include financial rewards, social standing, power, and "the
knowledge that one is performing some valuable social service." Second,
we need to determine institutional arrangements that will maximize the
efficiency with which the social good is achieved. Hodges uses medicine
to illustrate:

Thus, to take an obvious example, there exists a social need for health care. The medical profession is a particular social arrangement which is designed (well or badly?) to supply that need. The particular duties and obligations that are assigned to various members of that profession are by no means "writ in stone" and in fact there is constant pressure from within as well as without to change them in various ways. . . . All this is important to recognize because it focuses on the conventional and institutional nature of professions on the contractual view.

Hodges argues that neither the activity nor the contract model is an adequate basis, by itself, for professional ethics. His assessment of the difficulties of the activity view parallels Veatch's assessment in *A Theory of Medical Ethics*.[18] Both thinkers point out that the activity model lacks a necessary orientation toward the institutional nature of the profession and its foundation in general ethical principles, including a conception of social welfare. That is, the activity model is not responsive enough to the opinions, needs, and concerns of those outside the profession.

Veatch supports a contract theory of medical ethics. He calls it the "triple contract theory." It consists of "a three-level social contract or covenant that begins by establishing the most basic social principles for human interaction, progresses to establish a social contract between society and the professional group, and finally, provides a basis for individual contractual relationships between the professional and the lay person" (Veatch 1981, 110). Let us briefly examine each of these levels.

Like Engelhardt (whose thought we will examine in the next chapter), Veatch despairs of discovering a preexisting, universal basis for ethics. He thinks we must invent one. And, again with Engelhardt, he thinks we should invent one that everyone would agree on, given that we must come at the end to some kind of agreement. For Veatch, our moral convictions seem analogous to the pet theories of jury members. Each of us would, no doubt, like to legislate his or her own opinion. But this is impossible; there are too many moral convictions, too many pet theories. They cannot be harmonized. Just like jury members, we must come to some sort of agreement if we are to carry on with our business. Veatch rejects the idea that those who are strongest should coerce the others into adopting their view. He thinks that agreement of the sort desired has transcendental conditions. These conditions are the minimal conditions for a moral community. Veatch's next move distinguishes him from Engelhardt. Whereas Engelhardt holds that the transcendental condition for the possibility of a moral community is "mutual respect," Veatch argues for thoroughgoing equality.[19] Veatch's discussion at this point seems to be a replay of Rawls, and I will not discuss it here. Suffice it to say that where Veatch follows Engelhardt, he is susceptible to the criticisms that will soon be directed at the latter thinker. And, regarding the Rawlsian turn, even if we concede the need to invent a universal basis for ethics (Royce would not), it is not clear that any reasonable person, placed behind a veil of ignorance, would make the same choices as Rawls and Veatch. The reader of these thinkers likely learns more about the social and political orientations of these respective thinkers than about the decisions that all reasonable people would make under such conditions. I think that if Nozick were placed behind the veil, he would stick with his theory of entitlement. Royce would claim (with MacIntyre) that, apart from the viewpoint of one with a full gamut of actual purposes and desires, a workable concept of rationality or morality cannot be fashioned. Either the thinkers behind the veil would have these purposes, or they would have nothing to say. For instance, unless one values material wealth—by no means a universal value to all reasonable or rational persons—one will not be inclined to "bargain" for rights to material things.

The second level of Veatch's social contract is the contract between society and the medical profession. At this level we enter into the realm of medical ethics proper. We are concerned with "how health professionals might have special obligations and privileges not applicable to other members of the society." The obligations at this level and at the next "derive at least indirectly from the basic social contract" (127).[20] These obligations (and privileges) will arise, specifically, in an agreement between society and the medical profession, informed by the moral standards that are articulated in the basic social contract:

> Under this model the basic norms of a society are those that
> would be invented or discovered by people coming together to
> form a society from the moral point of view, that is, assuming
> that each person's welfare is taken fully into account. Within that

framework, the members of society might determine that special roles such as physician or patient should carry with them special rights and responsibilities. Some of those roles—what the sociologist calls achieved roles—one can choose to enter. Those who do can enhance their status from time to time by making a contract or covenant as a group with the rest of society. In that second contract or covenant the special norms for the role can be identified and made explicit. (130)

Veatch cites licensure as evidence for the existence of a social contract at this level.

The third level is the level at which patients and physicians make specific agreements. These agreements are bounded by the roles and obligations specified at the second level. But, within this framework, the physician and patient are free to establish by contract whichever ideals they mutually choose. The desirability of a contract at this level is predicated on the consideration that "If professional and lay persons can agree ahead of time on some of the constitutive elements of that relationship, neither will be forced into the intolerable situation of having to choose between violating one's conscience and violating the conscience of the other party" (136).

Veatch's triple contract theory has several major flaws. On the most general level, Veatch is susceptible to Hodges's objection against all contract theories of professional ethics. They neglect the manner in which professions generate their own internal goods and standards. Veatch exacerbates this problem by not recognizing how, at the second level, the social contract with society might grant substantial freedom for the medical profession to generate its own standards and to police itself. There are reasons to support such an arrangement, the foremost of which is that professionals will have a better insight into technical issues about enhancing health care than, say, politicians or attorneys. Veatch rightly points out that medical training and practice create a professional perspective that, on many important issues, diverges from the rest of society and therefore should not be trusted as the sole basis for resolving these issues. The same could be said of professional training and practice in politics, law, or ethical theory. This consideration does not eliminate the possibility that, on many issues, society will benefit the most if they leave clinicians to their own resources. Society could benefit from their expertise[21] as well as from the fact that it would not have to rely so much on external inducements to insure the integrity of clinicians. Physicians would be strongly motivated by goods internal to their practice.

Several other problems attend Veatch's notion of a contract between society and the medical profession. First, if there is a contract between society and medical professionals, then how can society justify reforming health care without approval from the medical profession? To reform the health care system is to modify the social contract. If this is done without approval from both sides, it is a breach of contract. Veatch says that physicianhood is an "achieved role" that is chosen. But what young physicians achieve and choose is far more vulnerable than goods secured by a contract. If we view the role of physician as something predicated on a social contract, then the physician is entitled to just compensation when the contract is modified against his will. There are, I believe, members of the medical profession who view their role in contractual terms. These doctors think that the eight or so years they spent in professional training (not to mention the grind of premedical studies)—accumulating debt, enduring long hours, and passing muster during several layers of formal and informal evaluation—have fulfilled their part of a vital bargain with society. Veatch would have to agree that their indignation about reforms (including many suggested by Veatch) is justified.

Second, he insists that, if a contract is moral, it must be negotiated from the "moral point of view" (i.e., behind the veil of ignorance).[22] This point needs to be defended in the face of the common perception that moral results can be obtained through a process of bargaining in which all parties represent their own peculiar self-interest. The legacy of this view dates back to Hobbes's contractarian theory. Veatch responds to this challenge, in part, by arguing that, due to asymmetries created by the natural lottery, bargaining for one's self-interest will not always have equitable results. What Veatch really needs to do is defend his view that thoroughgoing equity—even to the point of negating the individual benefit derived from inherited talents—is the goal of morality. If Veatch wants to wipe out every contract that is not fashioned from "the moral point of view," then he will wipe out, in one moment, the entire corpus of existing social contracts. From the viewpoint of a contractarian, this would seem to represent a return to the state of nature.

Perhaps the biggest flaw in Veatch's view is the idea that approaching the results that would be obtained by disinterested observers is possible (131). Recall the misgivings we have already expressed about the likelihood of achieving this end with respect to a basic social contract. These misgivings would be amplified in the case of bargaining about the contract between professionals and society. How are nonphysicians to understand the goods internal to the practice of medicine when they try to place themselves behind the veil? How could anyone understand the irreducible plurality of human responses to illness? Yet such an understanding would seem to be necessary if we expect to bargain equally for the good of all patients. In considering the issue of standards arising from our attempts to determine how those in the original position would view the contract between society and physicians, Veatch concedes that many will be arbitrary (132). If so, they are, by his view, nonmoral.

Regarding the third social contract, between physicians and patients, Veatch's requirements at the first two levels do not leave much room for sectarian concerns.[23] He has attempted to preserve individual choice in the context of specific arrangements between providers and their patients. Such arrangements "could include both lay people and professionals holding a common moral, philosophical, theological, or ideological framework. Christian Science, Jehovah's Witnesses, Seventh Day Adventists, holistic health centers, and Oral Roberts' medical complex in Tulsa are the ideal models of this, even if they have not chosen the right system of beliefs and values" (137). Unfortunately, within the context of the legal limits he would impose on the rights of physicians and patients to incorporate their own values into the clinical relation, the domain of individual choice becomes rather vacuous. For instance, consider the possibility that all the physicians in a city are Catholics, holding that abortion is immoral. Veatch would like to preserve their "right of conscience" by allowing them to exclude this practice in their contract with patients. Nevertheless, he suggests that society might make the access to abortions an essential element of its contract with physicians. It would seem that, barring a successful effort to transplant abortionists into the aforementioned city, these doctors would finally be compelled by government to violate their moral beliefs.

Royce would claim that both Veatch and Engelhardt commit the same fundamental error. They pass over the real basis of morality. Compare the following passages. The first is from Veatch:

If, without the benefit of having discovered a universal base for a common moral framework, one finds oneself in the unfortunate position of having to interact with physicians, nurses, health planning bureaucrats, patents, and others who make social medical ethical decisions, what is one to do? This is a world that, in Hobbes's terms, is nasty, brutish, and short. If one is to avoid the terror of a struggle of brute force putting all against all, it would be prudent to strike a bargain for inventing, if possible, some framework that provides at least a minimal basis for communal interaction. (Veatch 1981, 118)

The second is from Engelhardt:

To summarize the difficulty, in order to establish the authority of any particular moral perspective, one will need to establish the authority of a particular moral sense. Establishing the priority of any particular moral sense will require a moral sense to choose the right moral sense. One will have the same difficulty in the case of the selection of that second-order moral sense, and so on *ad infinitum.* (Engelhardt 1986, 38)

Royce would observe that both thinkers traverse a similar road to skepticism about universal moral ideals. They neglect to observe that, in the very process of inquiring (and expressing skepticism) about these values, they express an underlying, universal value—the need for a universal moral community, which is the basis for a common moral framework. Veatch correctly recognizes that this need arises out of the tissue of everyday social life. He notes that it would be prudent for everyone if we agree to establish a moral community. He does not, however, seem to recognize the monumental importance of this common human need. If we recognize that each prospective member of our moral community is someone who wants to establish an objective basis for moral ideals, then Engelhardt's infinite regress is stopped in its tracks. The authoritative, universal human value is discoverable. It is the need to establish a universal moral community.[24]

Royce might be attacked by these other thinkers for providing an inadequate basis for difficult decisions about the conduct of health care. He would probably respond by supporting a less restricted, more sectarian approach to the health care enterprise. Veatch insists that we need a common framework for dictating the basic responsibilities of physicians that runs across sectarian boundaries (113). But this opinion is based on the belief that a universal human community must be achieved instantly. Veatch thinks this demand can be met only with the Rawlsian social contract. Royce would be very wary of the "leveling" effect of such contrivances. He would argue that certain thinkers—namely those of a Rawlsian stripe—would therewith institute the hegemony of their own values (probably through some very forceful acts of coercion that, nevertheless, would be called "agreement" rather than "force"). In the process, the initiative and ability of individuals, as well as small communities, to articulate their own values would be stifled. Moral progress toward the goal of a great community would also be impeded. Ultimately, Royce would defend sectarianism in health care for the same reasons he defended provincialism. He would hold that the greater medical community should be the ideal of several separate, well-differentiated health care institutions. Each should cultivate its own special vision, always keeping in mind how its mission coheres with the missions of other medical institutions. Ultimately, sectarianism might disappear. But, if so, it is only because of a genuine convergence of these varying sects. Sectarianism would not be legislated out of existence.

Royce would maintain, of course, that medical institutions, of whatever variety, should be devoted to the ideal of loyalty to loyalty. He differentiated between wise provincialism and false sectionalism on the basis of this devotion and would make a similar distinction between wise and destructive sectarian models of health care. How Royce would conceive the role of government in impeding the development of destructive sectarian institutions is debatable. But it is clear that he would not sanction the imposition by government of the kind of broad restraints over the practice of medicine suggested by Veatch and Engelhardt. He would point out that such restrictions, far from establishing a spirit of community, would be more apt to elicit revolt.

Hodges recommends that we should regard the activity and contract models as complementary. To a point, I think, Royce would agree. There is utility, from a perspective informed by the ethics of loyalty, in preserving a role for contractual obligations. The need for viewing the practice of medicine as an activity would, of course, also be wholeheartedly acknowledged by Royce. But Royce would insist that physicians define themselves primarily as members of a greater medical community, rather than as members of a profession. He would subordinate the professional goods to the higher social goods. At the same time, he would insist that social obligations be internalized, as moral commitments, rather than legislated on the basis of a contrived social contract.

Medical ethics based on the philosophy of loyalty spans the interval between the divergent perspectives of professionals and their patients at the same time that it mediates the tension between the professional and the contract models of professional ethics. It provides a substantive basis for human and professional rights, preserving their relation to correlative commitments and obligations. It helps us overcome the tendency of viewing the interests of individuals as antagonistic to the interests of communities. And it teaches us that preserving the initiative of individuals is one of the surest measures for achieving the ultimate harmony that is the basis for every lasting human ideal. These qualities should become more evident as we turn, once again, to questions about the grand tradition in medicine.

6

❖

Revising the Tradition:
The Structural Criterion

W
ho is the loyal physician? If Royce is correct, this physician is a member of a community along with others who are loyal to the same cause. This cause consists by necessity of a rather complex set of ideals, which are to a large degree received from a moral tradition. We have described the greater medical community as the bearer of this tradition and as a community that commands the loyalties of its diverse members.[1]

In the final three chapters of this book I will attempt to give a theoretical account of the cause to which the loyal physician ought to be devoted and the virtues that this physician ought to cultivate. In this and the succeeding chapter, we will discuss of the medical tradition and how it ought to be reformed in accordance with Royce's philosophy of loyalty. In the final chapter, I will draw the elements of our discussion together into a brief summary of the ideal and the virtues of a loyal physician.

In what follows, I will keep the discussion general, except where specific illustrations seem helpful. Such generality is no mere concession to space but reflects the fact that Royce's notion of loyalty is not an abstract formula and is recalcitrant to its use as a premise for simple calculations. Achieving specific moral imperatives and policy guidelines, under a loyalist program, can occur only through an arduous, socially expansive process. Such imperatives and guidelines are not the province of a solitary commentator, except in the sense of someone who points suggestively ahead. I cannot overstate the importance of recognizing that this study is no cookbook. The more specific my recommendations, the more they will and ought to be open to revision from the perspectives of other practitioners.

Judging a Tradition

Royce offers three criteria for judging, and revising, a tradition. The first, which I will call "the structural criterion," appeals to the internal consistency of a tradition. To apply this criterion, one searches for incompatibilities within the tradition.

Incompatibilities within a tradition may be elementary or practical. An elementary incompatibility, as I will understand it here, is an incompatibility between general laws or rules that operate within a system. A practical incompatibility is an incompatibility between imperatives that are derived from general laws or rules. Incompatibilities of the above sorts are not strictly logical contradictions, since they are relations between rules and imperatives rather than between propositions. Nevertheless, I will refer to them at times as "contradictions," expanding the meaning of this term to include all forms of rigorous incompatibility. I use the term *derived* in a weak sense, to include relations that are less rigorous than entailment. Thus, it is possible that two or more mutually compatible rules may generate incompatible imperatives in practice. In such a case, we are often better advised to revise how we interpret a rule than to abandon or reformulate it. For example, someone may claim to derive the imperative *Tell Mr. Jones that I think he has lung cancer* from the rule *Be honest*; and the incompatible imperative *Do not tell Mr. Jones that I think he has lung cancer* from the rule *Do no harm*. In this case it is not clear that the rules are incompatible, because it might be possible for a clinician to be honest with Mr. Jones while keeping temporarily silent about the diagnosis, and it is also quite likely that, despite the initial pain, Mr. Jones would not really be harmed by learning of his clinician's opinion.

A second criterion for judging a tradition is what I will call "the moral criterion." It consists essentially of a question. Does the current form of the tradition aim at the realization of a great community? Recall that all ideals are expressions of purpose. To apply the moral criterion we must inquire about whether or not the purposes expressed in a tradition promote the purpose of approaching the great community, conceived in terms of the cultivation and the harmonization of loyalties.

This approach, of course, may be branded as a hopeless appeal to utopianism. To such a criticism I have two replies. First, Royce, though not straightforwardly a meliorist, views the attainment of a great community as occurring at the culmination of an endless process of change. As such, the goal (the "utopia" if we must) is a faraway destination, not a state of affairs that can be instituted in the short term through the right legislation or by inculcating the requisite virtues in the next generation of leaders and citizens. When approaching the great community, one will ask of each social custom whether it leads us toward or away from the great community. The question, Would this custom be a part of the great community? is not always relevant, as many of society's justifiable rules and conventions will surely become unnecessary or obsolete as humanity progresses to a higher level of moral life. The problem with utopianism is not that it pursues a remote vision but that the utopian mentality is often too wrapped up in a final vision, losing sight of the present. The utopian is characteristically unable to deal with the notion of an intermediary state, trying instead to establish the final goal at one fell swoop, cramming utopian ideals down others' throats. Such an orientation is not an effective agent of change, and utopians are thus often perceived as particularly impotent individuals.

My second response is simpler. It should not be surprising that a moral idealist such as Royce pursues ideals. And, insofar as his idealism is thoroughgoing, it should not be surprising that he views the universe in idealistic terms. If one is unsatisfied with the end result—with the notion of the great community—then one ought to attack Royce's basic arguments. I have not fully presented Royce's fundamental metaphysical theses or his theology. Nevertheless, I have argued for the establishment of an idealistic moral orientation as the only kind of morality that coheres with our experience of values. The possibility remains that human values are ephemeral, and, ultimately, lead nowhere. I will not try to convince the reader otherwise here. I do claim, however, that in order to engage in the moral life, one must assume that we, collectively, are headed somewhere and that where we are headed is an important matter. The justification for this claim is contained in my discussion of loyalty and the moral insight. It is there that critics of Royce should aim their attacks.

I call the third criterion for the evaluation of traditions "the practical criterion." With the first two criteria we examine the theoretical suitability of the tradition. With the third we examine its appeal. Does it motivate us? Will it stimulate our passion and spur us to action? These questions are as critical as any, and, quite possibly, the hardest of all to address.

The problems exposed by the application of these three criteria are, of course, moral problems. In the rest of this chapter we will look at structural problems. In the next we will look at problems arising from the application of the moral criterion. The third criterion will come into play in the final chapter.

There are two structural problems that arose from our discussion of the medical tradition in chapter one. First, there is the incompatibility between altruism and egoism. Second, there are incompatibilities generated by different interpretations of the obligations to respect the autonomy of patients and to promote their well-being. I will discuss each of these in turn in this chapter.

ALTRUISM AND EGOISM

One of the theses that Royce maintained and frequently reiterated throughout his career was that the alternative between the moral outlooks of altruism and egoism presents itself only at a relatively low level of moral comprehension. For Royce, the very use of these terms reflects an error. In his oft-repeated, but somewhat misleading, phrase "the illusion of selfishness," Royce portrays this error as being of the nature of an illusion.

When Royce speaks of the illusion of selfishness he is not claiming that selfishness is an illusion. He readily admits that some people are selfish. As we have seen, selfishness is the basic condition of those at the first level of moral life. The illusion of selfishness is, rather, an illusion had by selfish people. The "illusion of selfishness" refers to a characteristic moral shortsightedness of these persons. It is a kind of ignorance.

We know that Royce holds that every person has a psychological need to be loyal. We also know that this need is rooted in the need for establishing a personal identity. For Royce, the project of establishing a personal identity may be viewed as the vocation of each individual human being. Consequently, the cultivation of loyalty is considered to be each individual's most important commitment. At the first level of moral life, this commitment is viewed, as we have seen, as a personal task, where individuals proceed essentially on their own. At this stage, selfishness is natural. At the level of natural loyalty, the individual perceives personal ideals and personal identity as part of a higher unity—the unity of a natural community. No longer quite so selfish, our individual does not distinguish personal ideals from those of other members of the community but identifies personal well-being and the well-being of other community members with these unselfish ideals. Finally, at the third level of moral life, the individual recognizes that there is an ultimate unity of all human aims. This understanding is, of course, the result of the moral insight. Here the individual perceives personal moral destiny in terms of the progress towards an all-inclusive ideal, where each person's values intermingle harmoniously with those of others. Thus relieved of earlier shortsightedness, our individual can no longer be regarded as selfish and is no longer affected by the illusion of selfishness.

It might seem, then, that Royce argues for altruism and against egoism. This conclusion is correct if one defines altruism as the attitude of thoroughgoing and practical concern for the well-being of all persons, including oneself. However, so defined, altruism is not the contrary of egoism. Altruism of this sort, when it recognizes the great community as a unifying ideal, is a perspective from which egoistic concerns are harmoniously aligned with concern for the well-being of others. Altruism has also been defined as the pursuit of the well-being of others, to the neglect of oneself. By this definition, altruism is the contrary of egoism. It is the ideal of the self-denying self. Royce holds that such a perspective is as shortsighted as egoism.[2] Neither view recognizes the ultimate ideal, and both views inaccurately distinguish between the well-being of various individuals.

The underlying need for self-realization, harmony, and continuity, fulfilled only through loyalty to loyalty, is what stimulates every ideal, no matter how shortsighted the latter, no matter how unconscious the need. Thus, every ideal is an expression of the desire to be loyal to loyalty. Egoism and altruism (of the second sort above) thus reflect, for Royce, different responses to the same basic misconception. Both the egoist and the altruist fail to recognize an underlying unity between the ideals of all individuals. Thus, they make a distinction between their own well-being and the well-being of others, and they both feel compelled to choose between promoting their own interests or promoting the interests of others. The egoist chooses the former, the altruist the latter. Genuine loyalty, on the other hand, does not make this distinction and therefore cannot be described as altruistic or egoistic.

One should not infer from our discussion that we are all loyalists to the great community and that, therefore, all of our motives are morally admissible. The desire or need to be loyal is not loyalty. Loyalty is the will-

ing, practical, and thoroughgoing devotion to a cause. If we act from loyalty, we must be conscious of a tie between our intentions and a specific
service to some community. We must be aware of our ultimate purpose
to that degree. Insofar as we function at lower levels of moral life, many
of our motives are twisted manifestations of a mostly unconscious desire
to be loyal. We seek completeness but do not, at this level, understand
that we can be complete only through membership, through loyalty, in an
eternal community. Our intentions are vitiated by our lack of insight.[3]
Thus, morally blameworthy ideas are comparable to false ideas. In both
cases, our conception of what we mean is, ultimately, quite different from
what we actually mean. Loyal ideas are analogous to true ideas. Ideas that
express natural loyalties are analogous to ideas that express provisional
truths. Ideas that express genuine loyalties are more closely analogous to
ideas that express absolute truth, although, because our present ideas
about how to serve the great community issue forth from our imperfect
vision, they too are provisional in their details.

The tension between altruism and egoism, then, is not ultimate. It exists only from a limited frame of reference. This insight is important. But
the reader is probably quite aware that it does not entirely dispatch our
problem. We are, after all, limited, finite beings. And, except possibly in
our finest moments, we will still frequently experience the tug of selfishness
as an impediment to our nobler aspirations, or, on different occasions, experience the disintegration of our altruistic ideals as our energies and passions are depleted through self-neglect. The theoretical solution to the ego-
ism-altruism opposition leaves us, nevertheless, with a practical problem.

An approach to the practical problem is to recognize that egoistic and
altruistic interests are mediated by our conception of loyalty. This approach is, essentially, a practical application of the theoretical discussion
above. Our loyalties are imperfect. But they are, nevertheless, the highest
expression of our moral ideal, and, as such, the source of our moral obligations. When egoistic and altruistic concerns clash, we are therefore
obliged to mediate the clash through an appeal to our loyalties.

A paradigmatic example in the life of a physician is the tension between the desire to earn a high income and the desire to serve the public
interest by providing low cost medical care. Proponents of altruism would
claim that the latter interest should take precedence; proponents of egoism would likely choose the former.[4] To mediate this conflict, we should

recognize that (1) both desires represent interests of the medical community, (2) the desire to earn a high income generally also reflects the physician's loyalty to communities other than the medical community, and (3) the optimum balance between these interests is determined by an appeal to the great community. Let us consider each of these points in turn.

That the desire to provide low cost medical care coheres with the interests of the medical community is obvious. Aligning the physician's desire to earn a good income with the interests of the medical community, however, is not so straightforward. Three considerations in this regard deserve mention. First, the physician is a member of the community, and, insofar as his vision of service to this community includes the notion that physicians are professionals—persons who earn a living by their service to an ideal—the notion of remuneration becomes a matter of community interest. Second, paying clinician-interpreters is a sound strategy for implementing the objectives of the medical community. Recall that the ultimate ideal of the medical community is to fight illness. This objective will be realized much more efficiently if the clinician-interpreter spends a great deal of time and effort in mastering this role. But such an effort cannot realistically be expected from someone who is not a professional— it would be folly to think that we could enlist a competent corps of physicians in the manner that some communities enlist a volunteer fire department, by training persons in their spare time to function, on a volunteer basis, as part-time clinicians. Finally, how well physicians are remunerated will have an effect on parameters other than the cost of care. Two negative consequences would certainly result if physicians were not relatively well paid: (1) bright young individuals, with the talent to become good physicians, would lose some incentive to pursue the practice of medicine; and (2) physician morale would suffer and, predictably, the quality of care would likewise suffer.

One reason for an inevitable decline in physician morale that would correspond to a decline in income is the fact that physicians—like all individuals—have multiple loyalties. One of the most common of these loyalties is to the family. Physicians are apt to be concerned about providing amenities, especially a good education for their children. Suffering a loss of income would impede the physician's ability to serve this cause. It would interfere with the physician's loyalty to family. Many other such loyalties find expression, at least in part, through financial capacity.

To resolve the tension between the desire to earn a good income and the desire to provide low cost medical care by an appeal to the great community will involve several steps: (1) the mediator must examine how both desires reflect an interest of the medical community (as we have begun to do above); (2) the mediator must examine how each desire reflects the interests of other communities to which members of the medical community belong; (3) the mediator must compare these competing interests as impartially as possible, that is, from the best possible approximation of the perspective of loyalty to the great community; and (4) most important, the mediator must seek, through the aforementioned steps, to understand these so-called "competing" interests as expressions of the same ultimate purpose.[5] This final step is what most thoroughly distinguishes the loyalist from those engaged in the weighing of interests that characterizes ordinary decision making. The loyalist's method is to correlate various interests with a comprehensive, unifying vision of moral life and the moral community. There is, for the loyalist, no self-contained standard apart from this comprehensive one. How any individual executes such a procedure may vary; but each vision, each tentative resolution, represents an act of loyalty to the great community.

One of the caveats of undertaking such refined moral deliberations is the possibility of underestimating or neglecting the presence and influence of one's own moral vices. Specifically, I worry that physicians all too easily delude themselves into thinking that their desire for a high income is a manifestation of loyalty—backed by considerations such as we have already brought forth—rather than the embodiment of greed that it often is. Physicians—especially certain groups of specialists and subspecialists—often make far more than a "comfortable" life would require. Though I am in no position to announce the fitting, equitable and morally appropriate remuneration for any specialty, I think I would be remiss not to identify the morally nefarious reality of greed and its potential to afflict and overwhelm the medical community. Certain observations fuel my apparent pessimism on this issue.

First, organized medicine has often seemed to be more concerned with maintaining power, privilege, and financial security than with serving the greater medical community. Why, otherwise, would it have championed so many of the competition-limiting practices and regulations that we mentioned in the last chapter? Good evidence has never been available to show that the quality of physicians would decrease if a greater number of qualified students were admitted to medical school. In fact, common sense tells us the opposite. So, why are there so few positions? Some apologists would tell us that it is necessary to keep the number of medical school admissions down because a glut of doctors would actually lead to an increase in physician fees. This prospect would not apply, however, if there were not so many factors (supported by organized medicine) that artificially insulate fee structures from market forces. Allopathic medicine's treatment of nonallopathic alternatives has also, at times, reflected narrow self-interest more than loyal devotion. Has anyone ever demonstrated that patients with low back pain get better when they go to M.D.s than when they go to chiropractors? Within the fraternity of allopathic medicine, we find another inequity—the fee differentials between various specialties. Radiologists, for instance, earned a median income of $264,446 (for those in group practice) in 1994, compared to $122,000 for family practitioners.[6] Why are radiologists paid so much? Do they endure a harsher training environment than family practitioners? Not at all—in fact the opposite is the case. Is their day-to-day grind more demanding than that of family practitioners? Once again, the opposite is generally the case. Are they required to be smarter or to know more than family practitioners? Again, no. No other medical professionals exceed family practitioners in terms of the breadth of information relevant to their practice. Is the income differential between radiologists and family practitioners a result of impartial market forces, and thus fair in this limited sense? To a degree, perhaps. The general opinion in the marketplace seems to be that brief, minor procedures such as reading an X ray or removing a small skin lesion are more valuable than bedside diagnosis or the communication of medical information. Nevertheless, specialists seem to foment this notion when they limit the number of doctors who are trained and licensed in their specialty and when they collaborate on maintaining exorbitant fee structures, creating an artificial monopoly and the corresponding illusion that their services require a higher overall level of training and expertise than the services of generalists. I suspect that family practitioners are able to live quite well on their present incomes and are not to be pitied. Nevertheless, as a group, they may more closely embody our moral ideal than most other specialties, not merely because they place a lower priority on making a lot of money but also because of their organizational objectives, which clearly incorporate the notion of a moral community.

The second observation supporting my contention that greed is a real player in this matter suggests that the medical profession has done less to emphasize community service than a healthy ethics of loyalty would require. Given the manifold ways in which medicine is nurtured and supported by the larger community, we could expect a more solid tradition of medical philanthropy. Why do so few physicians see community service—perhaps as a brief commitment to the Public Health Service or the Peace Corps, or in terms of a regular volunteer work for community health programs—as a moral imperative or, simply, a nice way to enhance their lives? Could greed be a factor? This issue deserves far more attention, and is far more nuanced, than the purposes of this book allow. My point, for now, is that the tension between egoism and altruism reflects not merely the partial truths that are manifested at early stages of moral insight, but also a tension between good and bad habits—between virtues and vices—that will influence medicine's moral destiny. When egoism is fueled by greed, the potential for moral growth is diminished.

Egoism and altruism, we have concluded, should no longer be viewed as fundamental postures. Neither one should be expected of the physician, of the patient, or of scientist. Instead, each of the members of the greater medical community should be expected to be loyal to this community. Two sources of conflict will be allowed and expected: (1) members will also be loyal to other communities, and conflicts will arise between the interests of these communities and the interests of the medical community; (2) differences of opinion will arise about how best to serve the interests of the greater medical community. Whenever such problems arise, physicians must appeal to a conception of humanity's broader interests—i.e., to the great community. What we have, then, is the displacement of the version of morality that engendered the distinction between altruism and egoism—a conceptual shift that occurs when we move from one level of moral insight to another. Though we are not consistently able, as individuals, to view our values and the values of others on an equal footing, we will acknowledge that such a perspective is our ideal and that our moral obligation is to approximate the ideal as closely as possible.

AUTONOMY AND BENEFICENCE

The second structural problem that we have identified within the grand tradition in medicine is between respect for the autonomy of patients and respect for their well-being. I will refer to the theoretical formulations of these values, respectively, as the principle of autonomy and the principle of beneficence. To respect the autonomy of a person is to respect that person's freedom to make his or her own plans.[7] This freedom includes freedom of thought—to formulate one's own values—and freedom of action—to express or pursue these values as one sees fit. From our earlier discussion, we know that these freedoms are not absolute. It is impossible to construct moral values in isolation, and circumstances will always limit the possibilities we have for expressing them. Thinkers such as Cassell tell us that, given these limitations, we should view autonomy as consisting of two elements, authenticity and independence (Cassell, 1977). An authentic decision or action is one that is an expression of the ideals, habits, or motives we most consistently and consciously approve. An authentic action, then, is a genuine expression of will, attentive to a well-established purpose. Virtuous decisions and actions are authentic when they proceed from a firm and relatively unchanging character, approved by the agent. Actions that express vice may be authentic for the same reason. Decisions and actions are independent when they are uncoerced.[8] For our purposes, freedom and autonomy will be equated.

There are two ways in which freedom of thought and action is commonly understood: as a moral side-constraint and as a value.[9] Moral side-constraints are negative injunctions that moral agents must observe, without exception, in pursuing goals. Side-constraints may be more understandable if we give an example of a nonmoral one. In the game of football, for instance, an offensive lineman may not grasp the jersey of a defender. This holding rule is a side-constraint. The goal of the offensive lineman is to keep defenders away from the ball carrier. It is not his goal *not* to violate the holding rule; that rule is only a constraint he must acknowledge as he pursues his goal. Values are, of course, the goals that moral agents pursue. It is possible, as Nozick has observed, to value respect for freedom without recognizing that respect as a moral side-constraint (1974, 29). However, it is not possible, in my opinion, to recognize respect for others' freedom as a moral side-constraint and not to value it (as one does in the football example for a nonmoral side-constraint), since adopting a moral side-constraint is a strong form of valuation. It is possible, however, to recognize respect for the freedom of others as a side-constraint while holding that there are higher values, though this would commit one to maintaining the controversial position that value A is more important than side-constraint C, though one may not violate C in order to attain A.

Bearing all of this in mind, there are three sorts of views about respecting the freedom of others to which I would like to call attention: (1) freedom is a value that may occasionally be compromised for the sake of higher or different values, (2) freedom is a value that must not be compromised, and (3) freedom is the highest value, and it must not be compromised. Each of these three views has been urged, at one time or another, on physicians. A leading proponent of the first view is Edmund Pellegrino, of the second is H. Tristram Engelhardt. We see the third view in the early work of Eric Cassell.[10] I will, with Royce, support a version of (1).

Respect for the well-being of patients interferes with respect for autonomy when the best way to promote the overall best interests of the patient necessitates an abrogation of the patient's autonomy. If the patient's well-being is equated with the patient's personal freedom, there can be no conflict between beneficence and respect for autonomy. Such a view, however, is ridiculous. No one would choose a totally free life on Mars, where life would inevitably be short and miserable, over a relatively free life on a planet such as Earth, where one would be restrained, perhaps, only from burping in public or murdering his children. There are, no doubt, goods other than freedom.

More interesting is the question of whether a person's well-being can be identified with the *fulfillment* of what one autonomously wills. The argument that autonomy is the individual's comprehensive good is often based on the notion, as above, that merely *having* autonomous will is enough. If I am stuck on Mars, I may will to be free of poison gas. Thus, my greatest good—and my autonomy—now correspond with the fulfillment of this end. From now on, when we speak of respect for autonomy, we will refer to regard for the fulfillment of autonomous choices, rather than mere regard for the preservation of an autonomous will.

Let us turn, for a moment, to the case of Ragnar, who arrives by ambulance one evening at Podunk Regional hospital. He is attended by Dr. Chester, who is the sole physician on duty. The night is a busy one, and Dr. Chester is already attending several very sick individuals when Ragnar arrives. The emergency medical technicians (EMTs) explain that, apparently due to his feelings about a recent breakup with his girlfriend, the twenty-one-year-old Ragnar ingested thirty-five amitriptyline tablets. A friend called the 911 immediately afterward. Apparently the friend walked in just as Ragnar took the last of the pills. Ten minutes later, he has arrived in the ER. Ragnar is presently alert and oriented. His affect is normal. He appears to be calm. His mental status exam is normal. He denies physical pain. He has not vomited. He lacks the physical signs that attend overdosages of substances like amitriptyline, such as drowsiness, seizures, tachycardia (fast heart rate), or other heart problems such as QRS elongation, conduction blocks, or dysrythmias. He has, in fact, a totally normal physical exam. He tells Dr. Chester that he tried to discourage his friend from calling the ambulance and that he was brought to the ER against his will (though he did not struggle). He explains that his intention is suicide and that he has been committed to his decision ever since the breakup with his girlfriend three weeks ago. The delay was due to the fact that he had to put his affairs in order. Having done so and having secured a supply of drugs he knew to be adequate for the task, he proceeded with the suicide. He says that his life had been centered on a relation with his girlfriend since they were ten years old and that apart from her company his life is pointless. Dr. Chester knows that Ragnar's apparently stable medical condition will be transitory. Amitriptyline is emptied from the stomach very slowly, due to its anticholinergic properties, and the effects of an overdose are frequently delayed. He informs Ragnar that, barring treatment, his ingestion will be fatal. Ragnar understands but asserts that he wants to die. Ragnar starts to leave.

Before we go on, it is worth noting that, if Dr. Chester has Ragnar restrained to prevent him from leaving, he is, in one (very tenuous) sense, not interfering with Ragnar's autonomy. Ragnar is still free to think whatever he wants and to struggle against the restraints, to shout obscenities or threats at Dr. Chester, or to engage in whatever other actions he wants, under the circumstances. We could say in this case that Dr. Chester puts Ragnar in a different (restrained) environment but leaves him free to do and think whatever he can in this environment. Thus, the freedom of one in restraints is analogous to the freedom of one living on Mars. If the physical environment is given, and not considered to be a variable, then autonomy in both cases is potentially complete. However, in Ragnar's case the physical environment is a variable, one that is under the control of persons such as Dr. Chester, and this fact is a crucial distinction. We generally think that a solitary inhabitant on Mars is free because his constraints are the result of impersonal forces. Ragnar's constraints, on the other hand, though physical, are the result of Dr. Chester's actions. It is clear that if Dr. Chester restrains Ragnar, he has not respected Ragnar's autonomy in the sense, noted above, of showing regard for the fulfillment of Ragnar's autonomous choices. Once again, this kind of respect for autonomy is what is at issue in this book.

The preceding scenario is not common, but similar situations do occur. I have chosen it because I believe it is one of the few situations where respect for the well-being of a patient interferes with respect for autonomy. Ragnar's decision to commit suicide has been deliberate and reasoned. It is made autonomously. Using Cassell's terminology, it is both authentic and independent. It is authentic because it is a decision that reflects Ragnar's character—he is, or has been, above all else, devoted to his relation with his girlfriend. It is independent because it is a decision that Ragnar has made on his own, free from coercion, and, apparently, free from merely temporary spasms of grief. Dr. Chester, if he holds freedom as the highest value, or even if he recognizes respect for freedom as a moral side-constraint, must allow Ragnar to leave. On the other hand, if he values Ragnar's well-being above his freedom, he must detain him. Royce, I believe, would support the latter alternative. Let us consider why.

Characteristically, Royce would have us resolve conflicts between beneficence and respect for autonomy by an appeal to some higher, mediating principle. On a general level, he would ask: how do beneficence and respect for autonomy promote the interests of the great community? Respect for autonomy is important, as we have seen, because a fulfilling life is possible only when a person lives according to a plan that is chosen autonomously. Loyalists must choose their own causes, and they must decide the manner in which they will serve. Freedom therefore becomes an essential constituent of the moral life and also an interest of the great community.

But respect for autonomy would be important to communities even if freedom was not conceived, from the standpoint of individuals, to be an important good. The very ideals that define a community can be served effectively only when the autonomy of its members is respected. As I have explained elsewhere, Royce considers the cultivation of individual differences to be a hallmark of thriving communities (1994, 251–254). Just as a multiplicity of tools will heighten the probability of doing any job right, so will a multiplicity of individual talents and strategies enhance the likelihood that the ideals of a community will be realized. The community cultivates individual differences by respecting the freedom of its members

In summary, respect for the autonomy of others is an important service to the community in (potentially) two ways. First, it facilitates the realization of community ideals other than the well-being of community members (if there are such ideals). Second, autonomy is important to the well-being of community members. Assuming the well-being of community members is an ideal of the community, then respect for autonomy is a service to the community because it serves this ideal.

To say, as in the second point above, that respect for autonomy serves the community because it promotes the well-being of its members is to support the principle of autonomy with the principle of beneficence. If this were the only reason for respecting the freedom of others, there would, again, be no conflict between beneficence and the respect for autonomy. But to say that respect for autonomy is good for the community, even apart from a direct correlation to the well-being of the individuals whose autonomy is respected, prompts a consideration that falls outside the domain of beneficence.[11] I will argue that respecting autonomy as a community value—apart from autonomy's relation to individual well-being—will have different implications at different levels of morality. At the first or second level, respect for autonomy as a community value will engender obligations that are extraneous to the obligations derived from the principle of beneficence. If everyone operated at the third level, however, the principles of beneficence and autonomy would be coextensive.

My reasoning on this issue is relatively straightforward. From the perspective of the great community, every truly autonomous action will support the well-being of the community and of all its members. We have held that autonomy is constituted by authenticity and independence. An autonomous action is one that is undertaken without coercion for the sake of an ideal that expresses the authentic concerns of the agent. For the genuine loyalist, the most authentic concern will be the service of the great community, or loyalty to loyalty. Insofar as the loyalist has attained the perspective of the third level of morality (a perspective, the reader is reminded, that adequately interprets the moral experience of all human beings), the service of the personal ideal will benefit all other members of the great community, since it is also service of their highest ideal. If I undertake the treatment of a patient who is another genuine loyalist, my concern for my patient's autonomy is equivalent to my concern for the well-being of that patient. If my patient is genuinely loyal, these two will not conflict.

On the other hand, suppose my patient, like Ragnar, is not a genuine loyalist. Ragnar autonomously wills to kill himself. If I, acting as his physician, respect his autonomy, I must allow him to carry out his will. If I act on the principle of beneficence, however, I must treat him against his will. The difficulty hinges on two senses of the term *will*. In chapter 2 we distinguished between a wide and narrow sense of the term. *Will,* in the wider sense, we said, spans all our purposes and includes subterranean purposes not yet fully articulated but that affect us nonetheless. It is to this wider sense of *will* that Royce refers when he writes that our moral task is to bring our own wills to self-consciousness (PL, 14). *Will,* in the narrow sense, was described as "the attentive furthering of our interest in one act or desire against another" (OP, 368). This concept corresponds closely with what moral philosophers call 'intention.'[12]

When I claimed that autonomous actions are authentic expressions of an agent's will, and, later, when I claimed that Ragnar autonomously wills to kill himself, I used the narrow conception of *will*. Of course, at the first and second levels of morality, the autonomous will, narrowly conceived, will not always choose that which is most conducive to the overall well-being of the agent (since we have defined the well-being in accordance with the ideal that is willed in the wider sense). Thus, at these levels, there will be conflict between the principle of beneficence and the principle of autonomy. Of course, it would be possible to define *authenticity* by reference to the wider notion. In this case, loyalty to loyalty, being the ultimate principle of the will, would be the most authentic purpose of each person. I think that Royce would resist this move. The clinician who defines *au-*

tonomy in terms of the broader notion of authenticity adjusts the everyday meaning of this term to accommodate a Roycean theory of morality. In the process the clinician loses the practical advantages of making a distinction between autonomy and beneficence and is apt to foist private moral beliefs, en masse, upon the patient. A major reason for the ascendance of the principle of autonomy in biomedical ethics is concern about safeguarding the peculiar moral beliefs of each patient. The broad notion of autonomy is a useful theoretical tool, but to use it in the clinical setting would be to cancel out every objection to Roycean ethics in one stroke. Such a move would not merely antagonize the moral sentiments supporting the principle, but it would be incompatible with Royce's fallibilism.[13]

As a Roycean, I hold that Ragnar's deepest need is the need for genuine loyalty. I identify his welfare with the fulfillment of this need, rather than the fulfillment of his will (understood in the narrow sense). I cannot argue that because only genuine loyalty can harmonize the various disparate objects of his will, he really wills loyalty above all else. This would contradict Royce's claim that something is willed (once again, in the narrow sense) only if it is consciously chosen. Ragnar has not consciously chosen to be genuinely loyal. Royce would have us save Ragnar, against his will, because this action best serves to cultivate loyalty. If Ragnar lives, it is possible—even probable—that he will learn to value causes other than his doomed romantic relationship. He has already shown a capacity for devotion. Amidst the lonely wreckage of his thwarted relationship, there no doubt remains a spark of passion—for meaning and fellowship—that is Ragnar's human inheritance, and it can, eventually, ignite his love for another, greater cause. In his future, Ragnar is likely to reinterpret the failed romance as a stepping stone in his moral development. Death, on the other hand, would deny this potential outcome.

Ragnar's autonomy ought to be violated by Dr. Chester, ultimately, because Dr. Chester has good reason to believe that Ragnar's conscious will is not in harmony with his deeper, not wholly articulated, purposes, and that to allow Ragnar to kill himself is tantamount to allowing him to betray himself. Dr. Chester's move is presumptuous, and he therefore needs to be careful. Is he thrusting his own moral outlook into Ragnar's life? Is he destroying the only loyalty for which Ragnar is capable or inclined? These are troubling questions. Perhaps Ragnar is not destined to view the world through the lens of loyalty. Even so, Dr. Chester must presume that Ragnar is connected in some way with the larger community, and he must pause at the absence of this connection in Ragnar's current account of his life story. Something is amiss. On the one hand, if Ragnar has no ties with the community—including Dr. Chester—it is difficult to see how Dr. Chester has any responsibility for respecting Ragnar's autonomy. On the other hand, a sounder conclusion obtains if Dr. Chester opts to save Ragnar's life, with the well-grounded hope that something greater than lost romance can be made of it. To understand better why respect for autonomy cannot be supported outside a nexus of shared human values, characteristic of substantive human communities, it is worth looking at a thinker who believes that it can—H. Tristram Engelhardt.

Though Engelhardt maintains that building a community is a prerequisite to ethics, his minimalist ethical community, we shall see, falls short of providing the structure he needs. Let us summarize his program. First, he characterizes ethics as "an enterprise in controversy resolution" (1986, 39). He then goes on to argue that, of four possible modes of controversy resolution, only one is open to ethics. Force is not an option, because it is not an act of rationality, and ethics is, by definition, an affair of the rational intellect. Conversion and rational argument are not options because to succeed they must appeal to ideals that are not universal—Engelhardt cites the failure of the Reformation and Enlightenment projects as proof that we do not have access to universal ideals. Therefore, "the only remaining hope is resolution by agreement" (1986, 39–40). Next, he observes that "such agreement is either free or forced" and assumes that it is preferable for it to be free. From here, Engelhardt concludes that respect for freedom is a transcendental condition for the possibility of ethics (1986, 42). He recognizes that, in so doing, he establishes respect for freedom both as a side-constraint and as an ideal of moral communities (1986, 43–56). The moral community that defines itself in terms of the procedural principle of respect for freedom is, in Engelhardt's view, the most authoritative, but also the most content-poor, moral community—it "has the ability to span numerous divergent moral communities," but it lacks the full array of guidelines necessary to provide members with an understanding of the good life (1986, 54).

One of the great weaknesses of Engelhardt's position is that he has no basis for establishing that free agreement is better than forced. Although he claims that the resolution of first-order moral controversies (controversies about which specific activities are moral) must occur, by definition, through the employment of rationality and, therefore, through the application of higher-order ethical principles and not force, he cannot maintain, on this basis, that force is not a valid means of securing agreement on these higher-order ethical principles. The whole thrust of his argument against the resolution of moral controversies by sound argument amounts to the claim that there is no morally nonarbitrary basis for establishing higher-order moral principles. He cannot move consistently from this claim to the position that the (higher order) principle of autonomy is nonarbitrary. Nor can he say that it is the only possible means of securing agreement, since various forms of coercion are also possibilities.

Recall that Royce had two reasons for respecting autonomy. It turns out that, at the most basic level, Engelhardt has only one. Further, Engelhardt's rationale is circular. He arbitrarily chooses free agreement over forced agreement. Respect for autonomy becomes, on this arbitrary basis, the *only* ideal of his minimalist ethical community. Then, within the context of this community, he justifies the priority of respect for autonomy by pointing out that it is the community's defining ethical ideal. There is no other reason to respect autonomy because there is no other ideal. Because there was no good reason for establishing this ideal in the first place, the reasoning is circular.

Apart from the aim of loyalty to loyalty, the two possible ways of justifying the principle of autonomy—service to the moral community and beneficence—may diverge. This is where we find Engelhardt. He cannot justify his allegiance to the principle of autonomy by an appeal to beneficence because there is no foundation for beneficence in his authoritative moral community. He subscribes to a version of pluralism that contends that persons (or communities) are mutually isolated. It is, therefore, not surprising that he must appeal to the good of a higher-level, surrogate community in order to sanction his views about respect for freedom. Because he contends that the ideals of content-full moral communities are arbitrary from the vantagepoint of rationality (and, therefore, in his view, from the vantagepoint of secular morality), he must fashion a relatively contentless community. He achieves this end by defining his community in terms of a procedural principle, and, of course, this principle becomes the inviolable centerpiece of his moral philosophy.

It is interesting that both Royce and Engelhardt justify their moral philosophy on the basis of transcendental arguments. This is consistent with the fact that both thinkers recognize a substantial debt to Kant. Engelhardt defines moral life as the enterprise of resolving controversy peacefully and argues that respect for the freedom of others is a transcendental condition for the possibility of such an endeavor. Royce defines moral life as the intelligent pursuit of ends and argues that there are two transcendental conditions: reasonableness and impartiality. He then goes on to show that the rational individual will evolve through three stages of moral life that correspond with its increasing ability to extend the scope of its impartial reason—at the first level to the spectrum of its own thought-signs, at the second to the thought-signs of a community, and at the third to the thought-signs that compose the moral universe. Both thinkers demand respect for the freedom of others. But Royce demands much more and understands respect for the autonomy of individuals as a derivative of a higher devotion to the well-being of communities. If Engelhardt is to maintain his position, he must defeat Royce's arguments.[14]

There are at least three other problems for Engelhardt. First, he does not provide a sound-enough basis for his crucial distinction between "free" and "forced." If force is to be rejected, as Engelhardt argues, we must ask, To what degree? Should we proscribe only the infliction of physical pain or physical harm? Such a proscription will be difficult to define, as the boundaries between physical and psychical pain or harm are indistinct. Or, should we proscribe the forms of behavior modification that characterize so much of the early training of our children? Engelhardt frequently observes that infants and fetuses are not persons; he does not, however, give an adequate account of how they become persons and how the views they come to hold when they become persons are influenced by their models. In what sense do these educators and parents "force" individuals to hold the views they endorse? The boundary between coercion and freedom is fluid. This fluidity is highlighted within Royce's account of moral development and the moral life. Engelhardt, on the other hand, writes as if the boundary is distinct. It is incumbent upon him to show why.[15]

Second, Engelhardt's only arguments for rejecting an appeal to universal values are that (1) such appeals have thus far been unsuccessful, and (2) every value must be justified in terms of other values, which would lead to an infinite regress. The first of these arguments does not speak to Royce, the fallibilist, who expects a long succession of various degrees of failure before eternal and absolute values are discovered and agreed upon, but sees no reason why this prospect negates the attempt to pursue such values. The appeal to universal values cannot be called a wholly unsuccessful endeavor just because these values have not been precisely determined. Any physicist will admit that the universal laws of physics have yet to be precisely determined—Newton failed, and, presumably, so did Schrödinger and Einstein. I doubt that Engelhardt would call for the abandonment of attempts to discover and formulate the universal laws of physics. The second argument is unsound if values are self-legitimizing in the sense that we have explained in our discussion of the moral insight, and there is an ideal that harmonizes all values, as Royce has argued.

Third, Engelhardt never approaches a recognition of the moral insight, and he relegates virtues such as loyalty, gentleness, and temperance to the status of afterthoughts. Engelhardt proclaims that "tolerance is the cardinal virtue" (1986, 382). Tolerance, in Engelhardt's hands, is a rather blunt instrument. Understandably, he devotes little attention to it. Royce might want to point out that tolerance comes in only two varieties: (1) the habit of toleration of views and practices that do not directly or obviously harm the causes to which one is loyal, and (2) the habit of toleration of views and practices that do directly and obviously harm the causes to which one is loyal. Royce strongly agrees that tolerance of the first variety is important. It amounts to respect for autonomy. He would hold that tolerance of the second variety amounts to moral cowardice. When one's cause is violated, Royce believes that, as a loyalist, one is obligated to defend it.[16] Engelhardt, on the other hand, seems to support both forms of tolerance. He would advise us that we should not allow our moral commitments (except for the commitment to the principle of autonomy) to intrude into the affairs of our secular community. Such a view might result in controversy avoidance, but the community life that resulted from such a radical form of tolerance would likely be disjointed, shallow, and unfulfilling. The image of tolerance, in Engelhardt's hands, is a kind of milquetoast, the embodiment of moral apathy. For the aspiring clinician, tolerance of this sort provides very little in the way of a personality ideal.

With such paltry attention to the characteristics of the good practitioner, it is doubtful that his system would provide a very powerful impetus to moral behavior. That is to say, Engelhardt's ethics is not inspirational. For Royce at least, this flaw is important. It is a function of moral ideals, from his point of view, to fuel our passion. They are no mere final cause of moral life—they are its efficient and formal cause as well.[17]

In summary, the polarity between the principles of autonomy and beneficence is, for Royce, analogous to the polarity between egoism and altruism. In the context of moral life within the great community, the poles are joined. However, we do not currently live within the great community, and our aspirations to genuine loyalty are generally puny. We must deal with commitments to autonomy and beneficence that will conflict on occasion, just as we must deal, at times, with our selfishness. In both cases we must appeal to our ideal of loyalty to loyalty. When the two principles conflict, Royce has us adhere to the principle of beneficence. Beneficence, for Royce, is nothing other than the cultivation of loyalty in other persons. According to his view, no other justification exists for the principle of autonomy than this one.

The result for the medical tradition is that Royce would support an ethics of beneficence similar to the one portrayed by Pellegrino and Thomasma in *For the Patient's Good*. Royce and these authors share several important views: (1) they recognize a hierarchical supremacy for the principle of beneficence over the principle of autonomy; yet (2) they hold the principle of autonomy in much higher esteem than earlier proponents of paternalism (the view that clinicians exceed patients so drastically in knowledge of the concrete goods of health and illness that they will frequently be morally required to act without the consent or implied consent of a patient to benefit that patient); so that (3) they would severely restrict the possible scenarios in which one could act without the consent of a patient and not be blameworthy. Royce differs from Pellegrino and Thomasma by endorsing a different conception of the well-being of individuals. This point will come out in the ensuing chapter.

7

❖

Revising the Tradition:
The Moral Criterion

We have seen how two structural problems (in this case, elementary incompatibilities between general principles or ideals) would lead, under Royce's tutelage, to revisions of the grand tradition in medicine. Before we conclude, it should be worthwhile to consider how several moral problems would be approached by Royce, and the tradition, in consequence, further refined.

Recall that the moral criterion for revising traditions consists of an evaluation of how well they promote our progress toward the great community. The loyal clinician, along with loyal citizens, scientists, and politicians, will repeatedly ask of medicine's institutions, "How well do they serve our ideal?" Often we will be dissatisfied. In this section I will express some of the shortcomings I see in the grand tradition of medicine. Far from being comprehensive or authoritative, my observations and suggestions should be taken as the fruit of one individual's quest to honor the lofty standard of loyalty to loyalty. When I fall short, I ask the reader to consider that the errors are more likely due to my own personal shortsightedness than to a deficiency in the ideal of loyalty to loyalty.

I will begin the chapter by looking at several moral issues that hinge on the manner in which medicine is a profit-making enterprise. This topic will lead directly into a discussion about various forms of gatekeeping. From here, we will talk about the problem of balancing the need for focusing on technical expertise and competence with the need to view medicine within "the big picture," morally speaking. Our desire to understand patients as more than repositories of disease, amenable to technical interventions, will spawn a discussion of "narrative ethics" and of "the ethics of care." Both of these developments will be seen as potential allies of Royce's ethics of loyalty, but several potential pitfalls with each approach will also be identified. Finally, we will conclude by looking at how our Roycean theory shifts the boundaries of medical ethics beyond the traditional loci of sticky situations, patient rights, and moral rules.

MEDICINE AND ECONOMICS

In the May 2, 1994, issue of *Sports Illustrated*, E. M. Swift decries the fact that several athletic leagues for youth have banned the postgame handshake. Evidently, postgame handshakes have frequently become a forum for ugly and often violent displays of hostility or taunting. In several instances throughout the nation, league superintendents have opted to cancel the ritual rather than risk further violence. Swift blames adult supervisors—parents and coaches—for their failure to teach youths that sportsmanship is more central to athletics than winning: "Far better to keep the handshake and, if necessary, eliminate the games. Sit everyone down for a few weeks—cancel the season, if need be—until the players, parents, coaches, administrators, and fans get the message that sports are fundamentally unimportant except in the context of the values they teach."

Swift's article became the topic for several letters to the editor. Though most respondents sided with Swift, there was one outspoken critic, who responded as follows:

> Let's face it, winning and competition are the lessons of sports. Kids don't play sports to learn valuable lessons about life. Those lessons should come from school, church and the home. Kids play sports because they want to compete and experience that unequaled feeling of being a winner. What's the point of hearing your opponents say, "Good game"? It isn't a good game when you lose. Simply put, winning is the objective whenever people step onto the playing field. If it isn't, then why keep score?

The controversy is rather straightforward. Swift believes that the immediate aim of athletic competition—winning—is subsumed under higher aims, such as developing a sense of fair play, learning to cooperate, and learning that technical mastery is achieved only through dedication and practice. His detractor holds that only winning is important. There is no doubt about which side of this controversy Royce would choose. In fact, Royce firmly held that athletics have an important role in moral development. Though there would have been no questioning the postgame handshake in Royce's day, Royce nevertheless shared many of the concerns that we see today in Swift, and he foresaw many of the pitfalls that beset modern athletic competition. The following words from *The Philosophy of Loyalty* seem prophetic:

> It is the extravagant publicity of our intercollegiate sports which is responsible for their principle evils. . . . Fair play in sport is a peculiarly good instance of loyalty. And in insisting upon the spirit of fair play, the elders who lead and who organize our youthful sports can do a great work for the nation. The coach, or other leader in college sports, to whom fair play is not a first concern, is simply a traitor to our youth and to our nation. (PL 124)

Of course, our present topic is not the role of athletics in the development of youth. Swift and his objector are relevant to our discussion because their disagreement has an analogy in the world of business—where health care is a major player—and because Royce would mediate the business controversy in much the same way he did the athletic one.

There are many critics of ruthlessness and amorality in business. James Sheehy is one of them. His story, summarized by Shaw and Barry in their textbook *Moral Issues in Business*, is another reminder of our need to cultivate loyalty. Sheehy is a human resources manager from Houston who spent a summer working "undercover" at a fast-food restaurant owned by a relative. The great majority of his fellow employees were from middle and upper income families, many of them home from college for the summer. Shaw and Barry summarize his findings:

> What Sheehy reports is a whole generation of workers with a frightening new work ethic: contempt for customers, indifference to quality and service, unrealistic expectations about the world of work, and a get-away-with-what-you-can attitude. . . . Theft was rampant, and younger employees were subject to peer pressure to steal as a way of becoming part of the group. . . .

All that customer service meant . . . was getting rid of people as fast as possible and with the least possible effort. . . .

Sheehy's co-workers rejected the very idea of hard work and
long hours . . . they dreamed of an action-packed business world,
an image shaped by a culture of video games and action movies.
The college students in particular, reports Sheehy, identified with
the Michael Douglas character in the movie *Wall Street* and believed that a no-holds-barred, trample-over-anybody, get-what-
you-want approach is the necessary and glamorous road to success. (Shaw and Barry 1992, 177–178)

Sheehy, then, noted reprehensible behavior in aspiring businesspeople
that was similar to what Swift noted in young athletes. Imagine that
Sheehy had an opponent like Swift's. The reply might be something like
the following:

Let's face it, economic gain and competition are the lessons of
business. People don't sell food, build houses or practice medicine in order to learn valuable lessons about life. Such lessons are
the province of the home, the school and the church. People engage in business because they want to experience the unequaled
feeling of dominating competitors and accumulating wealth. If
profits are poor, business is a failure. What's the point of providing a good meal, of building a quality home, or of saving a life if
there is no profit? Simply put, profit is the only important motive when the fast-food operator takes an order, when the house-
builder raises his hammer, and when the surgeon dons his scrubs.
If it isn't, then why should they be paid?

Royce would be no more receptive to this kind of proclamation than
he would be to Swift's critic's. With so much of public life influenced by
business—not merely through business transactions, but also through the
effects of advertisements and corporate political lobbying—the attitude
expressed in the above passage would be disastrous to the aim of cultivating loyalty. Unfortunately, this way of thinking is common in American
business.

Royce's position on this issue is substantially shared by a modern
thinker, Paul F. Camenisch. Camenisch offers a threefold argument

against the notion that the only aim of business is the maximization of profit. First, he notes that not every profit-oriented enterprise is considered a business, citing bank robbery as an example because, as Camenisch notes, bank robbery is not concerned with the provision of goods and services. Second, he notes that, historically speaking, the provision of goods and services antedates the aim of accumulating profits. Profit making and capital accumulation, he observes, emerged as aims of human activity only because they became a necessary means for the efficient and satisfactory provision of goods and services. This suggests that the provision of goods and services is a more central function of business than making a profit. Thirdly, he argues that the very fact that businesses have flourished and continue to be accepted by society reflects the enhancing effect they have had on social welfare.[1]

Camenisch concludes that businesses ought to be judged on the basis of their contribution to the human condition:

> All three of these ways of addressing the relation between these two elements would seem to confirm my position that the provision of goods and services can, perhaps must, be given priority over the profit element in our understanding of business. The major implication of this position for the resulting business ethics would be that the assessment of business as such and of specific business enterprises would begin with the question of whether the goods and services produced thereby serve to enhance or detract from the human condition, whether they contribute to or obstruct human flourishing. Implicit here is the suggestion that businesses engaged in producing goods and services which do not contribute to human flourishing are engaged in a morally questionable enterprise, and those engaged in producing goods and services inimical to human flourishing are engaged in immoral activity. . . . (Camenisch 1992, 256)

This recommendation, of course, echoes Royce's. But whereas Camenisch is not ready to offer a theory about how we can define human flourishing, Royce offers the ideal of loyalty to loyalty. Royce would hold that businesses ought to be evaluated by the same standard we use to evaluate human individuals. Loyalty is the supreme human good. The propagation of loyalty is the measure of human flourishing. Businesses, like human individuals, ought to cultivate loyalty. The good ones are the ones whose loyal activities have the overall result of cultivating and harmonizing loyalties. The corporation or other business organization, large or small, is properly a kind of community. As we have seen, every community must have ideals. Morally acceptable ideals are ones that have been fashioned to serve effectively the ideal of loyalty to loyalty.

Business activity, then, should not be merely a profit-oriented enterprise. It should be loyalty enhancing. This conclusion is consistent with what we have already said regarding the physician as businessman. Though we have maintained that there is a basis in the philosophy of loyalty for the view that physicians ought to be well remunerated, the ideal of remuneration or profit was subsumed, in our discussion, by higher ideals. This appraisal, as we have seen, runs counter to a popular account of the businessman as one whose occupation is the pursuit of profit. I will call such an account the "entrepreneurial model." The entrepreneur, it seems, is one who identifies himself more as a seeker of profit than as a specially qualified provider of goods or services. Because of the relation between capitalism and the entrepreneurial model, a question arises. Is capitalism to be eschewed by the loyalist? Or, more specifically, should the medical community reject free-market models of the provision of medical services?

Royce never addressed either of these issues at length. It is plausible that Royce's opposition to the concept of rugged individualism and his recommendation that provincial communities occupy themselves in co-operative ventures such as the beautification of the community are evidence that he rejected bare-boned *laissez faire* capitalism. On the other hand, Royce is careful to indicate that competition is no impediment to the spirit of loyalty, as long as it is not the kind that delights in the total destruction of the opponent. Perhaps he would condemn today's corporate raiders. But I believe he would approve of wholesome economic competition, resulting in improved goods and services, and of the moral improvement of the competing parties. Royce selects athletics as a paradigm for this constructive form of competition (PL, 123–124; RQP, 229–287). In economic life, as in athletics, too much concern with the bottom line leads to a loss of focus on higher ideals.

Since Roycean ideas about the proper role of business are not widely accepted, I think it is dangerous for health care professionals to look at themselves primarily as business people. But, recognizing that the provision of health care is a form of economic activity, and an expensive one at that, I believe that a Roycean critique of medical economics may be valuable. Two major recommendations about the way medicine does business seem to be in order. Each represents a revision of medicine's tradition, or in the way the tradition has come to be interpreted by many.

The first recommendation has already been mentioned but needs considerable fleshing out. Royce, I believe, would recommend that the medical community aim at reversing a modern trend toward industrialization. By "industrialization" I mean the process by which organized medicine becomes more and more a profit-oriented enterprise, concerned with matters such as advertising, avoiding liability, and lobbying on behalf of the financial interests of medical professionals. No doubt, these matters warrant some attention. But I find it distressing that, as a practicing physician, my intercourse with organized medicine is dominated by issues of liability, remuneration, health care reform and cultivating a public image, while discussion of scientific medicine, and how best to promote the health and well-being of our patients, seems to be occupying a progressively smaller portion of our attention.

A glance at the Table of Contents from a recent ACEP *Products and Services Catalog* is illustrative. Of four periodicals, only one—*The Annals of Emergency Medicine*—deals with scientific investigations and clinical advances (and it also contains a large proportion of material that is dedicated to nonclinical matters). Two—*Foresight* and *Patient Transfer News*—are wholly dedicated to legal issues; and the fourth—*ACEP News*—is a newsletter concentrating on political issues. ACEP also markets several books: one is on marketing emergency services; one is on personal financial planning; one is a guide to state legislation; two books are listed that deal with coding and reimbursement; two are listed on contract management; and there are two books on legal medicine, one being the 438-page *Emergency Medicine Risk Management: A Comprehensive Review*, sold to ACEP members at the reduced price of $110. Altogether, the books on nonclinical topics outnumber the clinical ones.

I find the same trend when I sort through the plethora of brochures for continuing medical education opportunities that find their way into my mailbox. Everywhere there are seminars on coding and reimbursement, avoiding lawsuits, and effective marketing. Most of these "opportunities" are accredited to satisfy CME (continuing medical education) requirements. Once finishing initial training, a modern emergency physician can, quite possibly, maintain state licensure and remain an ACEP member in good standing without ever spending a minute in the study of clinical medicine. This physician can satisfy every requirement by learning about law, management or marketing.

Because most emergency physicians—even the so-called "independent contractors"—are laborers for profit-oriented businesses, they likely come under pressure to become knowledgeable about aspects of medicine affecting the bottom line. Frequently, this knowledge has little to do with promoting the well-being of patients. I suspect that for many clinicians there is little time left to devote to the scientific literature.

Even the current emphasis on "customer service" has its sinister side. Two very different ways of viewing quality medical care present themselves: (1) as a loyal service and (2) as a financially valuable product. For Royce, the first of these reasons clearly overshadows the second. The medical entrepreneur, in contrast, discards the first reason entirely. Customer service is important, in this latter view, because of its relation to the bottom line. Patients, as "customers," are often dehumanized. They are part of the formula by which the practitioner earns a living. Treating them well is important only because such treatment will enhance the practitioner's reputation and guarantee prompt remuneration without the threat of lawsuit.

Corresponding to the different reasons for providing quality medical care are two differing reasons for adhering to moral standards: (1) because it maximizes profits and (2) because the standards are important in themselves. Royce holds that a moral code (conceived as a framework of ideals rather than as a mere compendium of rules) is the embodiment of one's life plan; without it, our lives are meaningless. Abiding by the code is far more important than maximizing profits. The entrepreneur may also hold that moral standards are important, but only for the first of the above reasons. Because there is no deep attachment between the entrepreneur and his moral code, he will have no qualms about violating the code when he is sure the violation will not have an effect on profits. Just like the young athlete who is obsessed with winning and will cheat if he is sure he will not be caught, the entrepreneur is apt to be led into immorality whenever it seems to be a profitable affair.

The susceptibility of the entrepreneur to corruption is exacerbated when, in the course of conducting business, the knowledge of the consumer becomes dramatically inferior to that of the seller or provider. Of course, medicine is just such a "business." And, unfortunately, members of the health care industry have on occasion been guilty of disingenuously parlaying the ignorance of their consumers into enhanced profit (Burton 1994; Pollock 1995).

Whenever clinicians or their agents cultivate unwarranted dependence, they damage the cause of loyalty to loyalty. This sin, I believe, is also manifest in many current policies impeding the licensure of nurse practitioners, physician's assistants, and practitioners of alternative forms of medicine. No medical doctor can adequately defend the view that nurse practitioners or physician's assistants are not competent to manage the minor illnesses for which they are trained. Yet, lobbyists representing organized medicine have frequently sought to bar these practitioners from acquiring state licenses, often with arguments that would be laughable to an audience of honest, well-trained physicians. Further, some physicians have written off practitioners of alternative medicine—for example homoeopaths, acupuncturists, and chiropractors—without scientifically investigating their methods. The motivation for these positions is too often financial. In the end, patients are the losers because they suffer reduced options for affordable medical care. Doctors lose also, because their integrity is compromised.

The pharmaceutical industry, viewed by most as an element of the health care industry, has frequently been egregiously guilty of taking advantage not only of the ignorance of consumers, but also of the ignorance of doctors. Many such transgressions have come to the attention of the public. The tendency to discourage the use of generic drugs, for example, is frequently based more on "good business practice" than on good scientific evidence (King 1996). Further, add campaigns directed to the attention of physicians are often one-sided or polemical, focusing on data that support the use of an expensive drug while neglecting unsupportive data.

Insofar as a given physician is an entrepreneur, that physician is not a professional. We have defined the entrepreneur as one who, first and foremost, seeks a profit. A professional, on the other hand, is one defined largely in terms of service-related activities. The profiteer will practice medicine as the means to an external goal. The good life for the profiteer is composed of activities that lie outside the province of medical practice. The purpose of medicine is to provide the financial resources for these valuable activities. The professional, on the other hand, practices medicine primarily according to the view that this practice is part of the good life. For the genuinely loyal professional, the good life is the life of devotion to the great community, expressed, at least in part, through professional activities that are viewed as a service to humanity.

Ultimately, medical entrepreneurs are doomed to the same fate as the hero. Because such entrepreneurs measure the value of life according to a standard of worldly success, they are at the mercy of events. If health care delivery is reformed so as to make their specialties less lucrative, or if, God forbid, scientific developments so enhance the health of the public that their specific brands of medical service become obsolete, they are failures.

One of the negative consequences of the entrepreneurial approach to medicine, and the corruption it engenders, is the increasing government regulation of medical practice. Two factors invite regulation. One is the perception that some good or service is of fundamental value to human welfare and therefore ought to be available as a matter of right. This perception is the basis of the notion of a "right to health care." Obviously, health is high on the current list of human values. Another factor is the perception that the providers of some good or service are corrupt. It is the role of government, at least as it is now conceived by a large number of Americans, to see that important services are fairly and conscientiously provided to all citizens. If the medical tradition comes to endorse the entrepreneurial model of medical practice, it invites government regulation because the greed engendered by this model is viewed by the public as a corrupting motive and as a barrier to the equitable provision of health care.

I think the loyal physician ought to resist government intrusions. My reasoning on this matter rests on several considerations, especially on my views about the importance of preserving the autonomy of both providers and patients. Several bad consequences result from the involvement of government in health care. First, there is the problem of bureaucratic inefficiency. Much has been said about this seemingly intractable problem. The hassles associated with Medicare and Medicaid registration and reimbursement are infamous and do not bear repetition here. Workers' Compensation paperwork also is frequently trivial, redundant, and time consuming. And while physicians and nurses have labored over the multitude of tasks that are necessary to transfer a patient legally under COBRA (The Consolidated Omnibus Reconciliation Act), many stable patients, who could otherwise have been quickly transferred to a higher-level facility, have deteriorated. When regulations about who should be seen, where, and for what are formulated by individuals untrained in medicine, the resulting chaos is anything but conducive to efficient medical care. This concern is so ubiquitous as to be almost tiresome. I will not deal with it at more length now, except to acknowledge that, indeed, the issue is important, and, amazingly, many politicians still fail to take account of it.

In the chapter 1, I have already alluded to an important concern that does not always get the attention it deserves. Government tends to contradict itself. Often, it will require mutually incompatible actions. The classic case in the state of Tennessee may be the one created by the incompatibility between COBRA and TennCare. Suppose young Camille has a wart on her back. She decides, for whatever reason, to take her problem to the ER. Her physician will be in a bind. According to TennCare, the physician should refer Camille elsewhere—probably to an office provider—because she does not suffer from an emergency condition. On the one hand, if Camille is logged in, has her vitals taken, and sees the physician, the hospital will be penalized by the state of Tennessee (the hospital will not be reimbursed for the expense). On the other hand, according to COBRA, Camille must be evaluated by a health care provider before she can be sent away (which would include logging-in, vitals, history, and exam). If Camille is *not* logged in, does *not* have her vitals taken, and does *not* see a clinician, the hospital will be penalized by the federal government (its Medicare status could be terminated, and it could be heavily fined, or even sued by Camille). The contradictions engendered by government regulations are apt to confuse patients as well. Take, for instance, 1994 Tennessee House Bill Number 250 concerning reimbursements for ED evaluations. "Abdominal pain" or "pain from duodenal ulcer" are not on the list, while "appendicitis," "duodenal ulcer, acute with hemorrhage and/or perforation," "acute appendicitis," and several other specific emergency diagnoses are included. How is the patient with a duodenal ulcer, who has experienced a worsening of pain, to decide whether or not to go to the ER? The patient should go if the ulcer is bleeding or has perforated. Unfortunately, few patients can determine this on their own. These sorts of dilemmas have been engendered by legislators who lack expertise in medicine and who frequently do not even know the extent of their own laws. It is instructive that when Robert Williams, the past president of the American College of Emergency Physicians, met with the president of the United States to discuss health care reform, he expressed concern about COBRA. Alas, neither the president, nor his advisors, had heard of this legislation.[2]

A third reason for avoiding government control of medicine gets to the heart of the matter. Royce would maintain that both clinicians and laboratory researchers should be scientists. To assure progress in the medical sciences, he would hold, both clinical and laboratory events should come under the purview of the inquiring intellect. Royce acknowledges, along with Peirce, that inductive scientific generalizations depend on a fair sample (RLE 260). A fair sample, of course, is one that is comprehensive in the dual sense of covering as many situational types as possible and including the greatest workable total number of events. If a fair sample is important, then it is also important for medical research that the experience of as many clinicians and laboratory workers as possible contribute to the sum total of data and theories that are critically analyzed. It is, therefore, important that clinicians from every practice scenario be reflective and contribute their insights to the group.

If medicine cultivates such a spirit of inquiry, its treasury of hypotheses (both in technical biomedical science and in purely practical matters) will be multiplied in quantity and quality. Advances will accumulate more quickly in every aspect of medical technology and the provision of care. This advantage should not be difficult to apprehend. It can be highlighted by a consideration of the process of hypothesis formation and the factors that drive it. Royce identifies two types of hypotheses: (1) those that are directly testable and (2) those that are not. The first type of hypothesis is the one young students learn about in the study of induction and the scientific method. As Royce and other pragmatists stress, the formation of such hypotheses demands an important prerequisite—the apprehension and formulation of a problem situation. Dewey writes that "To see that a situation requires inquiry is the initial step in inquiry" (Dewey 1977, 34). If we are to respond to the problems of everyday medical practice, we must first perceive these problems and then articulate them. Presumably this task is better accomplished by those on the front lines—clinicians and patients—than by politicians or academicians. We made this same point when we noted that the chain of interpretations that constitutes the unfolding of medical knowledge always begins with the patient and must travel through the clinician before it reaches the research laboratory.

The same considerations apply to the second kind of hypothesis— what Royce calls a "leading idea." A leading idea is a regulative principle used to guide research. It is usually too general to be directly tested but receives indirect support when it leads to fruitful research. Royce uses Virchow to illustrate both types of hypothesis. Cited as an instance of the common variety is Virchow's hypothesis that all cells are descended from others. However, when Virchow claims "that diseases are not autonomous organisms, that they are no parasites which take root in the body, but that they merely show us the course of the vital processes under altered conditions," he is putting forth a leading idea (RLE 264). Of course, both of the aforementioned ideas have been immensely fruitful.

Leading ideas, I would maintain, must also be the province of both the community hospital or clinic and the academic center. Like simple hypotheses, they too are dependent upon the apprehension of a problem situation. Further, they demand uncommon creativity, initiative, and breadth of vision. The academician who assumes that these qualities are housed only in the university medical center is guilty of hubris, an unjustified and counterproductive form of self-confidence. He need only consult the annals of medical history to identify his error. Private physicians without university affiliations, such as John Hunter, have contributed some of medicine's most important leading ideas.

Hunter pioneered the study of inflammation. His initial investigations were spurred by his own experience with a torn Achilles tendon. Eventually, he inoculated himself with the organism that causes syphilis and observed the progressive stages of inflammation in this disease. Hunter developed the leading idea that inflammation—the process by which affected parts are healed—is the central aspect of disease. Nuland remarks that "To the present day, all over all the world, the most sophisticated methods of modern technology are being used to continue the investigation of inflammation that was begun by John Hunter more than two hundred years ago. The two treatises, on venereal disease and inflammation, became prototypes of clinicopathological description and of research in physiology, respectively" (Nuland 1988, 186). Both Virchow, with his idea about the alteration of vital process under pathological conditions, and Cabot, with his development of the clinicopathological review, are in Hunter's debt.

There is another reason that nonacademic experience is important to the integrity of research—because only here, at medicine's doorstep, are patient populations uncontaminated by referral bias. For researchers to assume that the characteristics of patients presenting to tertiary care centers mirror those of patients seen in primary care settings would be to commit the grossest fallacy in the art of determining the parameters of clinical problems. Nevertheless, this fallacy seems to lurk amidst the conclusions of a number of clinical investigations (Brody 1992).

What does all of the detail about scientific investigation have to do with the topic of government intervention? It is my contention that government involvement in the provision of health care will have deleterious effects on the quality of biomedical inquiry. These effects accrue through several mechanisms. First, the prospect of judicial oversight leads to an exaggerated concern with the formulation of clinical standards and adherence to consensus. We currently see this trend at work in issues such as the treatment of otitis media (middle ear infection). It is the current standard of care to treat any adult patient diagnosed with acute otitis media with antibiotics. This approach has led to an annual total (direct and indirect) cost for otitis media of about $3.5 billion. The practice is interesting in view of the fact that antibiotics have not been clearly shown to be of benefit in these cases. In fact, there is evidence to the contrary. For instance, a recent large international study showed that adults treated with antibiotics had a *lower* clinical recovery rate at two weeks than those who were not. Further, a history of prophylactic antibiotic use was isolated as an independent predictor of poor outcome (Bartelds 1993). Though the data have not been quite as impressive with children, there is still overwhelming evidence that the majority (approximately 86 percent) of children with otitis will not benefit from antibiotics (Bukata 1994). There are, no doubt, a multitude of reasons why physicians routinely continue to prescribe antibiotics for otitis media. Some of these reasons have clinical merit. Some that lack clinical merit still have nothing to do with government intervention (for instance, many patients, especially in the U.S., expect or demand antibiotics). However, I believe there are two important factors relating to the persistence of this practice that pertain to the role of government. First, physicians have gotten out of the habit of thinking through clinical issues, and instead often thoughtlessly appeal to the habits of their colleagues. Second, physicians fear legal consequences if they abide by their own better judgments, because the legal system holds adherence to the standard of care in higher esteem than adherence to sound clinical reasoning.

The first factor—thoughtless appeal to convention—has, I believe, largely developed because of the second. The net result is that, because of the fear of government reprisal, physicians are being taught not to think for themselves. Physicians are becoming, more and more, laborers with fixed job descriptions. The supply of thoughtful, scientifically oriented clinicians is dwindling. This trend should continue if government continues to play a major role in overseeing the conduct of clinical medicine.[3]

Researchers could relate a similar account of the effect of government oversight on their occupation. It seems that many Washington bureaucrats are seized by rather uninformed opinions about medical research, often due to the polemical influence of special interest groups. Good examples are the popular ideas that the medical establishment has not attended to research concerns related to AIDS or women's health. That AIDS has been the object of an overwhelming amount of medical research is obvious to anyone who cares to review the history of the disease. Claims to the contrary are generally so perverse or factually inaccurate as not to warrant comment. The situation with women's health is different. Even reputable, generally objective, publications such as *Scientific American* have published emotional and highly polemical pieces about the neglect of women in medical research. The fact that some of the claims of this camp are legitimate obscures the fact that many of their points rest on a disingenuous manipulation of the facts. Marguerite Holloway, in *Scientific American* (August 1994), claims that breast cancer, among other women-specific health complaints, is neglected in comparison to male concerns. She somehow fails to acknowledge that funding from the National Cancer Institute for research on breast cancer has long exceeded that for any other malignancy, though breast cancer presently kills fewer women (and men) than lung cancer. In 1996, breast cancer is expected to kill 44,000 women, while prostate cancer will kill 41,000 men (Parker et al. 1996). But breast cancer receives more than four times as much funding as prostate cancer (Kadar 1994). The fact is, no research on any male-specific complaint receives even close to the same funding as research on breast cancer. Further, both cancer of the cervix and cancer of the uterus receive more funding per fatality than prostate cancer (Kadar 1994). Women's groups have decried the fact that only 13.5 percent of NIH research (1987) was devoted to studying diseases unique to women. What they, and reporters such as Holloway who draw upon their rhetoric, neglect to mention is that only 6.5 percent of NIH funds were used to study uniquely male afflictions.[4]

When the machinery of medical research comes under the control of ignorant bureaucrats and selfish special interest groups, the quality of medical care is bound to suffer. It is no more morally defensible that policy be determined by these sources than that it be determined by the selfish interests of entrepreneurs within the health care industry. In fact, the latter source may be preferable. Indeed, Royce recognized the possibility of innovation springing from enlightened industrial self-interest:

> The sources of useful leading ideas seem to me to be various. Social, and in particular industrial interests, suggest some of them, as the perennial need of paying the coal bills for the steam engines suggested, as we have seen, one of the leading ideas which pointed the way towards the modern theory of energy. (RLE 266)

Even if my recommendations against the entrepreneurial model of medicine were rejected wholesale, forces within the health care industry would still be a more desirable source of leading ideas than government. The financial success of health care enterprises is dependent largely upon their ability to serve the public. When a genuine problem arises, the company or group which responds most effectively to it will succeed. In this way, the attentions of the private business sector remain concentrated on real issues. The make-believe world created by some special interest groups for the consumption of government policy makers is not so apt to intrude.

The trend of my discussion should be clear. I am supporting the more traditional, capitalist economic system while rejecting the appeal to self-interest that underlies many traditional versions of support for this system. I advocate a form of wholesome competition that has a basis in Royce's philosophy of loyalty, and I agree with several modern moderate political thinkers who believe that government intervention should be a last resort, instituted only when loyal service has given way to predatory entrepreneurialism.

My preference for capitalism does not, as the reader may now be thinking, mean that I support a return to the way we did medicine before the topic of health care reform came to the fore. The loyalist, I believe, should be as critical of that system as of the prospects for regulation through the hand of government. For one thing, twentieth-century American medicine has not been based on a free market economy. The medical profession has frequently done everything in its power to stifle legitimate forms of competition. I have already mentioned several of these maneuvers, such as lobbying for licensing standards that squash competition from practitioners of alternative forms of care. Other attempts to escape the legitimate pressures of a free market system would also likely be condemned by Royce.

Under the current tradition, patients are forbidden from obtaining relevant information about prospective physicians. They are not allowed to learn of the wound-infection or mortality rates of their surgeons. They have no access to information about the board scores or malpractice history of physicians. Further, patients are legally forbidden—largely due to the efforts of the medical establishment—from obtaining many relatively harmless medications without a prescription. Does it make sense that virtually anyone can purchase a chain saw or a .357 magnum but that people with sore throats are not allowed to purchase home streptococcal tests or penicillin tablets? And, of course, nonphysicians are generally forbidden to prescribe or dispense these goods.

Each of the examples in the preceding paragraph illustrates the phenomenon of interference with the autonomy of patients. The medical establishment has argued that preventing patients from choosing a physician is an important breach of liberty. I think Royce would agree. But he would also point out that preventing them from choosing alternative forms of medical attention and preventing them from learning to treat themselves, and from acquiring the resources to treat themselves, are also breaches of liberty. These abrogations of liberty are especially detrimental to the cause of loyalty because loyalty depends on free association. The health of the medical community, as I have noted above, requires the loyalty of patients as well as clinicians and researchers. But if we expect patients to be loyal, we must take care that their membership in the medical community is uncoerced. Loyalty is a *willing* devotion to the interests of a community. It is unlikely to occur in the case where patients have no recourse but to visit a certain provider. On the contrary, such an arrangement, especially when combined with the stifling presence of other forms of government regulation, breeds an atmosphere of distrust and litigiousness.

Several of these issues have been overlooked by mainstream proponents of increasing the autonomy of patients. Perhaps this is because many of these thinkers are supportive of extensive government involvement in health care. For example, a lot of pressure has built up to institute government oversight in matters of informed consent. However, now that informed consent has become a legal rather than a moral issue, the preoccupation with informed consent has vitiated overall concerns about the autonomy of patients. For instance, patients about to receive a lumbar puncture are often not allowed to exercise the option of not listening to all the gruesome details of what might occur in that one-in-ten-thousand case where something goes terribly wrong with the procedure.

Overall, then, we have offered four arguments for limiting the role of government in medicine. First, government intervention breeds bureaucratic inefficiency. Second, government regulations tend to contradict themselves. Third, government control stifles scientific inquiry. And fourth, important patient liberties are often undermined by government regulations.[5] It seems that the grand tradition in medicine, much like the tradition of several big businesses, has been influenced, on the one hand, by a policy of supporting government intervention whenever that benefits the rather narrowly conceived best interests of physicians and, on the other hand, by a policy of rejecting the hand of government whenever these interests are not maximized. This waffling support of the free market would not be approved by Royce. No doubt, Royce *would* agree that government intervention is sometimes necessary—especially in instances where a lack of scruples and an asymmetry of power have combined to create significant dangers for the consumers of fundamentally important goods and services. Royce would not acquiesce to natural rights arguments for the radical elimination of government intervention, such as we see in Nozick's theory of entitlement. Nevertheless, because of the considerations put forth above, I believe that loyalists should be committed to a limited government and to a capitalist economy. The medical tradition should be modified, along the lines suggested above, in this direction.

On the topic of medicine and economics, three other questions clamor for attention. First, what is the role of the HMO or other large corporation in the delivery of health care? This issue is, of course, particularly important, given the continuing political ramifications. I also believe that it is beyond the scope of this essay to consider it in detail. Nevertheless, a few comments are in order.

I do not believe that Royce would reject out of hand the notion of a role for the large nonprofit corporation in medicine.[6] In the absence of government interference, such corporations could be expected to respond reasonably to patient needs. But I believe that certain aspects of the gatekeeper function that such corporations may assign to primary-care physicians are morally objectionable. Specifically, I think that restricting access to subspecialists by requiring all patients to be screened by a primary care specialist is not generally justifiable. However, I doubt that this practice would persist in the absence of certain market conditions (for instance, the relative costliness of subspecialists' services compared to the services of generalists) that are largely the result of excessive regulation. Though I personally agree with the common opinion that better medical care often results when patients see a generalist than when they go straight to a specialist, I do not agree that access to specialists should therefore be limited. If patients decide they want to see specialists, then so be it.

Another important issue that I will not be able to consider in detail is the problem of providing medical care for the indigent. I think Royce would support efforts to achieve universal access to basic health care, though surely not because of any appeal to natural human rights. It has been and should continue to be a moral standard for all physicians not to refuse lifesaving or other emergent medical care to persons who are unable to pay, whenever this care can be provided without abrogating other significant moral obligations. Such an attitude is conducive to the cultivation and harmonization of loyalty. Further, it seems plausible that the government should be able to assist in the provision of health care by providing adequate welfare benefits. Citizens could be expected to use their welfare benefits to purchase private health insurance (or a portion of these benefits could be directly deposited by the government into the health insurance plan of their choice). The details of such a system would be complex, however, and are beyond my scope.[7]

Mention of the physician as gatekeeper brings up one more important issue dealing with medicine and economics. What role should the physician take in the apportionment of costly medical procedures and therapies? This issue has important implications that transcend the economic ones. It will be worth our while to consider it in some detail.

Gatekeeping

Pellegrino and Thomasma recognize three different gatekeeping roles. The first they call "de facto gatekeeping." It consists of a duty to order, suggest, or prescribe only those measures that the physician believes will be effective and beneficial. Pellegrino and Thomasma rightly consider this to be a traditional gatekeeping role and have no objections to it. Though I largely agree with their analysis, it is my opinion that the physician is often assigned too much power as a traditional gatekeeper. An example of how this power is overextended is the aforementioned unavailability of over-the-counter rapid strep tests and penicillin.[8]

Another kind of gatekeeper is what Pellegrino and Thomasma call a positive gatekeeper. Here the physician functions almost as a salesman, to *increase* the demand for medical goods and services in order to enhance profit. Pellegrino and Thomasma point out that "When positive gatekeeping is employed, the dependence, anxiety, lack of knowledge, and vulnerability of the sick person (or even the healthy person) are exploited for personal profit" (1988, 180). We have considered this type of gatekeeping function in our discussion of medical entrepreneurism. We rejected it for reasons similar to those cited by Pellegrino and Thomasma.

The most interesting and important form of gatekeeping is what Pellegrino and Thomasma refer to as "negative gatekeeping":

> In the negative version of the gatekeeper role, the physician is placed under the constraints of self-interest to restrict the use of medical services of all kinds, but particularly those which are most expensive. A variety of measures is used, each of which interjects economic considerations into the physician's clinical de-

cisions and limits his discretionary latitude in making decisions. (1988, 176)

They identify DRGs (diagnosis-related groups) as one form of institutionalized gatekeeping.[9] HMOs and PPOs (preferred-provider organizations) are others. If they had written their book later, they might have noted government-sponsored capitated systems such as TennCare. Many of the details of these systems are unimportant for our discussion. But it is needful to understand that each system functions on the premise that providing financial incentives to physicians to limit services will result in a desirable level of cost containment, with the minimum sacrifice in quality of care. There are two major ways in which services are limited. The first way we have already discussed. It is the method of limiting access to subspecialists through the utilization of generalists for screening purposes. I have already expressed qualms about this practice and will not discuss it further.

The second method of negative gatekeeping is to offer financial incentives to physicians to order fewer diagnostic studies and to employ less expensive therapies. I will call this procedure "negative gatekeeping of resources" and abbreviate it "NGR." The Roycean analysis of NGR differs from that of Pellegrino and Thomasma. Their respective accounts provide a natural centerpiece for the discussion of important contrasts between these thinkers and Royce.

Pellegrino and Thomasma think that NGR exacerbates two sorts of potential conflict: (1) the conflict between the physician's concern for financial self-interest and the physician's concern for the well-being of patients and (2) the conflict between the commitment of the physician to society and the commitment to patients. Both these thinkers and Royce want to avoid these conflicts, but they envision somewhat different ways of circumventing or mediating them.

Pellegrino and Thomasma take us back to ancient Greece in order to set the stage for the first of these conflicts:

Socrates, in his dialogue with the cynical Thrasymachus, was forced to admit that the physician was engaged in two "arts"— the art of medicine, which had as its end the health of the patient, and the art of making money, which had the physician's self-interest as its end and did not, in itself, contribute to the patient's welfare at all. (1988, 173)

They hold that this conflict is unavoidable, and that we can only hope to mitigate it:

> This de facto conflict of interest is difficult or impossible to eliminate, given that physicians must earn a living, support families, and have access to the same material goods as others. What mitigates the conflict is the ethical commitment of the physician to the patient's good, that is, to the principle of beneficence. (1988, 174)

They argue that NGR exacerbates this conflict by systematically exploiting it for the purpose of cost containment. The physician is able to maximize profits if and only if maximal limits are imposed on services. Thus, the physician's commitment to the good of patients is blunted.

Royce would observe that there is something strange about the notion of mitigation (or mediation) employed by Pellegrino and Thomasma. Essentially, what Pellegrino and Thomasma have ordained is that a conflict between A and B will be mediated by an appeal to B. How, we must ask, can an appeal to one of the conflicting parties justly resolve a conflict? Royce would want to mediate the conflict between A and B with an appeal to some C that recognizes the legitimacy of both A and B. "C," in this instance, would be the greater medical community. The commitment to the welfare of the greater medical community, in turn, will be mediated by a higher commitment to the welfare of the nation, and, ultimately, to the great community, as we discussed in chapter 5.

Of course, Pellegrino and Thomasma would claim that Royce has only displaced the conflict. The physician's commitment to his or her patient now conflicts with the commitment to social welfare. There are several ways in which Royce would meet this challenge. The first we have already considered. There should be, ultimately, no significant conflict between serving the individual and serving the larger community, since the very genuineness of the association between the physician and patient depends on a mutual commitment to a shared social ideal. The very possibility of mutual benefit between patient and physician depends on their inclusion in a larger community. When Royce mitigates the conflict between the interests of the physician and the interests of the patient by an appeal to such a larger community, he reinterprets these interests in light of a mutual ideal. I will not recapitulate the lengthy discussion of this matter, except to say that Royce is more thoroughgoing than Pellegrino and Thomasma in rejecting the common, but faulty, assumption that a pluralism of cultural and individual ideals undermines that unifying commitment to higher ideals that defines the pluralistic community. As we have commented on several occasions, Royce believes that the quest to realize social ideals is always strengthened when there is a diversity of opinions about how those ideals are realized.

Another way of meeting the challenge from Pellegrino and Thomasma is to explore the practice of triage. Royce would argue that the very existence of triage underscores the priority of social commitments over commitments to individuals taken in isolation. If I am seeing Mr. Starr for a sore throat, and learn that Mrs. Starr (whom I have never met) just arrived with crushing chest pain, I will leave Mr. Starr and attend to his wife. My decision will be based on the fact that a social interest is served by temporarily discontinuing my service to Mr. Starr. Public health is better served if we make a policy of seeing chest pain before we see sore throats.

Pellegrino and Thomasma would point out that I have undertaken the care of Mr. Starr, and have committed myself to *his* welfare. He is my patient. When Mrs. Starr arrives, she is not yet my patient. These thinkers, to be consistent, must hold that I am busy with Mr. Starr and therefore should not undertake service to Mrs. Starr. To avoid this unsavory position, they might want to argue that, since Mrs. Starr is present in my clinic and desires care, she is my patient. Also, since she stands to gain or suffer considerably, depending on my decision of whether or not to set aside temporarily my concern for the health of Mr. Starr, I should attend to her first. The problem here is that the only things that distinguish Mrs. Starr from the rest of the population are (1) that she is currently in urgent need of care; and (2) that she has sought my help. The first consideration surely does not qualify her as my patient. There are many persons across the globe who are in urgent need of care, and if I considered each of them to be my patient, then my obligations to them would be inexhaustible. People like Mr. Starr, with nonurgent conditions, would not stand a chance of ever getting my attention. Does the fact that she seeks my help qualify her as my patient? I would say that it does not. The physician-patient relation is based on freely taken mutual commitments. If individual physicians are required to attend to any patient who requests or demands their services, then they are no better than slaves, and, further, they are apt to become so overburdened that they will become of no use to anyone. Neither Pellegrino and Thomasma nor Veatch would deny that the physician who is overburdened with responsibilities should have the right to limit the number of patients accepted into his or her practice. Even the ED physician is expected to enlist the aid of colleagues when things get too hectic, rather than assuming personal responsibility for every patient who appears at the doorstep.

Yet I believe each of these thinkers would want to claim that, since Mrs. Starr's complaint is urgent, I am obligated to serve her. I cannot see any other basis for this opinion except the notion of a covenant, contract, or commitment to the general public. Preferring Mr. Starr's treatment over Mrs. Starr's is an example where the appeal to the health of an established patient interferes with a broader devotion to the public. Such is a case where the policy of localizing commitments purely within established physician-patient relationships seems clearly immoral. I am obligated to Mrs. Starr because she is a member of the medical community to which I am loyal.[10] I was obligated to her before she explicitly sought my services. My obligation to her is greater than my obligation to some other patient across town in another clinic only because I am in a better position to help her, not because I have any special contractual or moral obligation to her that I do not have to the other patient.

The fact that Mr. Starr would presumably prefer that I attend to his wife rather than continuing to care for him illustrates the previous point that, once any loyalist has committed to a community, that individual will not perceive the interests of others within the community to conflict with one's own in any substantial way. The husband-wife relation is a common form of smaller community, where the mutual devotion that is the ideal of larger communities is more frequently realized. It is not difficult to see, in this scaled-down model, how an individual can maintain his or her own distinctness, opinions, and personal style while rejecting the notion that his or her own self-interest is at odds with the interests of the marital community taken as a whole.[11]

Royce, then, would have a different way of understanding and formulating the tension between serving the health of individual patients and the interests of the medical community. But would his opinion about NGR differ significantly? In the long run, probably not. Royce would be wary of NGR for several reasons. Like Pellegrino and Thomasma, he would disapprove of the implicit credence it lends to the entrepreneurial model of medical practice. He would point out that, under such a system, the selfish physician would have ample opportunity to act in ways that benefit neither his patient nor the greater medical community.[12] He would also acknowledge that, given the imperfections in both physicians and patients, such a system would be bound to create or exacerbate mistrust. Pellegrino and Thomasma would agree on each of these points.

I believe that the aforementioned free-market approach to medical services would eliminate most of the problems that NGR is formulated to solve. One of the reasons that NGR is deemed to be necessary is that patients generally do not have any concern about the costliness of the care they seek. In general, they will choose even the most expensive procedures, if they think there is any chance of benefit. If the financial burden of medical care could be transmitted to the patient, so that the cost to the patient correlated with the cost to society (even granted that most of the costs would be footed by the social group as a whole, generally in the form of insurance), this tendency could be mitigated. Market forces would come into play, and the gatekeeping function would be performed by patients or, on occasion, by insurance companies, but not by doctors.

The available strategies for achieving this result are numerous but generally fall in line with the free market model. Whatever the course, it must involve a change in the tax laws so that persons who purchase their own health insurance, and those who choose high deductibles, are no longer penalized. Of course, optimally speaking, patients will be concerned with costs because they loyally respect community welfare. The loyalist program would be designed to inculcate this kind of attitude. Without it, Royce would maintain, our situation is ultimately hopeless. Nevertheless, such loyalty is not likely to become widespread in the near future.

I conclude that if we structured medical care in a Roycean manner, there would be no significant use for NGR. But, if we assume that the current trend of increasing government control will continue, and positive measures such as the widespread use of medical savings accounts are not implemented, I believe that NGR must have a place and would be supported by Royce. If patients are granted a "right" to medical care that is not conditioned on any correlative obligation, then the obligation for restricting the magnitude and expense of this care must come from somewhere. It can come from government, or it can come from the medical profession. If it comes from government, it will be based on inexperience and special interests. This fact is recognized by politicians who advocate the role of the physician as gatekeeper.

One of the virtues of NGR is that it checks the tendency to order and carry out unnecessary tests, therapies, and procedures that characterizes medical entrepreneurs. Presumably, the standard of practice would be divested of excess baggage. Worthless measures would be abandoned. This result, I believe, would have an immensely beneficial long-term effect for patients. The current obsession with obtaining medical care, which boarders on a national neurosis, would be mitigated, and eventually persons would seek care only for those conditions or symptoms for which medical care offers some benefit beyond the mere reassurance that one has been "seen by the doctor." Further, harm done through unnecessary measures would be decreased. I believe this result is evidenced in Great Britain and other European countries that regularly employ NGR. While massive bureaucratic inefficiency and paralysis have rendered those systems an impressive reason for rejecting government control, the fact remains that physicians in those countries have critically assessed the merit of therapies and procedures that American doctors long took for granted, with the result of improved care both in these countries and in our own (since our physicians read their literature). The European situation also illustrates the inculcation of saner general attitudes among laymen about the need for health care.

It could also be argued that NGR is beneficial because it countervails the tendency to practice defensive medicine. The problem with this argument is that, as we have seen, the benefit is accomplished at the expense of creating a double bind for physicians. In effect, government creates a problem (by creating expansive legal liabilities for physicians and by sanctioning a legal system that dramatically inflates rewards for medical malpractice), and responds to the problem by creating contradictory legislation. It would be better if physicians and patients together monitored the goals of the clinical encounter, working together to keep costs reasonable.

To summarize, Royce would probably join with Pellegrino and Thomasma in discouraging the practice of nontraditional physician gatekeeping, but his emphasis and his reasoning would be somewhat different. Ultimately, the differences between these thinkers hinge on the fact that Royce recommends that physicians subordinate devotion to patients to loyalty to the ideals of higher-level communities (in the rare instances where there is a genuine tension between these two). Because they have not fully developed the notion of loyalty, Pellegrino and Thomasma portray the physician in terms closer to those of the self-denying self than does Royce.[13] Another difference between the Roycean physician and the one portrayed by Pellegrino and Thomasma is that the former is first and foremost a citizen of the world, whereas the latter's self-concept is almost entirely that of a provider of medical services.

COMPREHENSIVE VISION

In 1936, Richard Cabot summarized an important attitude of doctors in a book designed for ministers:

> The central point in the doctor's makeup is *concentration* with its strengths and weaknesses. He is trained to focus on disease. . . . Concentration on diagnosis absorbs him so fully when he is with the patient that he gives little thought to the patient's life, character, and interests. Much he intentionally disregards. . . . What a lot there is that he does not notice, or even seem to notice! Yes, but so it always is with intense work. There is a good deal that a juggler does not notice while he is doing his tricks. Think how much a fox-hunter ignores when he is jumping a fence. We approve of his narrowness of vision because we can see what he is doing, but the doctor's furious activity is largely invisible. It goes on in his head or in brief, rapid, technical language quite opaque to the patient. . . . The doctor's strength is in the minuteness and accuracy of his work within his own chosen field. His weakness is in the crowd of obvious facts which he disregards, often rightly. (Cabot and Dicks 1936, 45–46)

Though Cabot's contemporary, William Osler, warned of entanglement in "the meshes of specialism (Osler 1932, 137)," Cabot's words reflect the consensus of his day and stand as a rather obvious prelude to the development of specialization in medicine. They also illustrate a formal recognition and endorsement of an important phenomenon that affects professionals of all varieties—what Michael Davis has termed "microscopic vision":

> What is microscopic vision? Perhaps the first thing to say about it is that it is *not* "tunnel vision." Tunnel vision is a narrowing of one's field of vision without any compensating advantage. . . . Microscopic vision resembles tunnel vision only insofar as both involve a narrowing of our field of vision. But, whereas tunnel vision reduces the information we have available below what we could effectively use, microscopic vision does not. Microscopic vision narrows our field of vision only because that is necessary to increase what we can see in what remains. Microscopic vision is enhanced vision, a giving up of information not likely to be useful under the circumstances for information more likely to be useful. . . . (1992, 49)

Davis goes on to explain that microscopic vision is not nearsightedness or myopia, since it is possible to look up from what one is examining microscopically and see what other people see. Microscopic vision is no defect in visual ability at all. It is a power. But, like most powers, it can be dangerous. The danger occurs when it is overutilized. "Real professional myopia is probably rare. Few professionals seem to lose altogether the ability to see the world as ordinary people do. Common, however, is a tendency not to look up from the microscope, a tendency unthinkingly to extend the profession's perspective to every aspect of life" (1992, 49).

Davis argues that microscopic vision is a common cause of professional wrongdoing. Professionals become so caught up in their specialized ways of viewing the world and evaluating situations, they fail to perceive nontechnical factors that should have important bearings on their behavior.

A classic example is that of futile medical treatment. Intensivists are trained to carry out elaborate multisystem analyses of their critically ill patients and orchestrate the harmonious employment of a huge variety of technically complicated measures designed to correct abnormalities discovered in their analyses. This process requires a capacity for the most powerful kind of microscopic vision. Unfortunately, due to the huge demands that such multisystem analyses impose, the intensivist is apt not to look up from routine work and factor in data that do not require the acuity of professional vision but which are, nonetheless, fundamentally relevant to the intensivist's mission. Thus, great amounts of time and resources are occasionally thrown into practices that only prolong the suffering of patients who are clearly at life's end, with no hope for meaningful recovery. A cynical term has emerged within the milieu of intensive care medicine to describe the paradoxical situation in which normal laboratory values have been restored but in which the patient nevertheless has not returned to any kind of humanly desirable existence—the patient is described as "euBOXic." Such episodes are tragic, and they are morally wrong. The intensivist, shorn of professional accouterments, would more readily recognize the inhumanity wreaked by dehumanized medicine.

In chapter 1 we talked about the tension that has developed between the notions of thoroughness and moderation. We remarked that, under the influence of thinkers such as Cabot and Osler, thoroughness came to be viewed as a kind of virtue without excess. I believe that this attitude developed because the emphasis on technical competence resulted in too much educational preoccupation with developing students' microscopic vision. Cabot and Osler themselves were probably not frequently guilty of such an excess in their personal practices. But they set the ball rolling with their effect on medical education.

There is one more issue I would like to address before we finish our discussion of comprehensive vision. That is the ideal of growth. As I have earlier commented, one of the differences between Royce and Dewey is that Royce is less likely to view growth as a good in itself. It is noteworthy that Cabot, though a student of Royce, tends to be more like Dewey on this issue. In Cabot's view, "Growth is the production of novelty within the range of a purpose and *without* dominant self-contradiction. Degeneration is the same thing *with* dominant self-contradiction. Learning, experimenting, admiring, sharing, and enjoying exemplify growth" (Cabot 1933, 453). Of course, Royce would generally be in favor of growth, as Cabot defined it. As we have mentioned on several occasions, Royce thinks the proliferation of different forms of knowledge and different experimental models is usually a boon to the community, enriching shared experience as well as the prospects for realizing community ideals. And Royce would agree with Cabot's contentions that "men have always needed and always will need to learn" and that "the duty to learn and the temptation to stagnate will collide again and again" (Cabot 1933, 7–8). But he would have serious reservations about another claim of Cabot's:

> When we find that our plans need improvement if they are to live in a changing world and to fit our changing needs, we come to recognize how unescapable is our need of growth, the central need of man. . . . Our desires are then seen to be good when they are in line with the authoritative need to grow, bad when by self-deceit they diverge from it. (Cabot 1933, 15)

Cabot has jumped from the legitimate recognition that growth is sometimes a moral requirement to the unwarranted conclusion that growth is an authoritative need. On the one hand, growth is surely necessary when it is required to serve the aims of loyalty. On the other hand, it should have no authority at all apart from these aims. Cabot, when he uses growth as a criterion of right and wrong, treads outside the philosophy of loyalty.

Though Royce would praise Cabot for stressing that growth, as a species of moral progress, must be viewed as occurring "within the range of a purpose," he would oppose the notion that the only means of progress is through increasing novelty. Royce differentiates two notions of progress: the first is accretion—the process by which things become more complex, without regard to a central purpose; the second is moral progress, where a state of affairs more conducive to the attainment of such a purpose is attained (WI II 421–423). Unlike Cabot, Royce recognizes situations where moral progress occurs without growth.

I submit that Cabot's moral preoccupation with growth was a factor in allowing him to endorse the proliferation of medical technologies without expressing caution about possible deleterious effects and without asking searching questions about when these technologies should be applied.

Royce offsets the tendency to deify thoroughness or growth with the philosophy of loyalty. Instead of advising professionals to view themselves as advanced technicians, concerned principally with microscopic details, Royce demands that these details be harmonized within a comprehensive vision of community life. Professionals must ask where their services fit into the greater scheme of things. And their perceptions of this greater scheme must be organized around the ideal of loyalty to the great com-munity—not to an abstract notion of growth. According to this view, technical thoroughness clearly becomes a virtue of the classic Aristotelian variety. It stands between a deficiency and an excess. The deficiency might be called cursoriness. The excess is futility, the quality of beating a dead horse. There is no reason that the loyal life should be prolonged beyond the stage where loyal service is still a possibility. The physician who acts as "the guardian of human life" in such situations is disloyal to humanity, diverting human energies and resources away from higher callings and as-saulting the dignity of his human subject.[14]

We have indicated that the provider is obligated to view his patient as more than a medium of pathology or potential pathology. There are things besides the objective determinants of disease that have important bearings on the patient's medical good. Ultimately, of course, we must ap-peal to the causes that the patient serves. How does a given illness relate to the loyal life of the patient? When momentous decisions about the manner and objectives of therapy are to be made, it is important that the physician be advised of these personal matters.

Examples abound. If a physician's patient is a dedicated father who has worked for years to see his daughter graduate from college, the physi-cian should be more inclined to suggest measures to prolong life and lu-cidity until the graduation date, despite effects that would be considered barbarous or inhumane in patients who had no such culminating event in their future. Perhaps the patient is a woman who is dedicated to caring for an invalid husband or child. She has a small osteosarcoma of the femur, discovered incidentally when she presented with a knee injury. The tumor is stage IIA—confined to a small section of bone, not affecting the cortex and not having metastasized to regional lymph nodes. But it is only mod-erately well differentiated, which means that it is likely to grow rapidly. The safest recommendation for this tumor is aggressive surgical manage-ment—the amputation of the affected limb at the hip. There is another possibility, however. The tumor could be excised locally, with an accept-able margin, after chemotherapy. Then a bone replacement procedure could be employed, such as cadaver allograft or metallic endoprosthesis. The latter approach is more risky, with a higher five-year mortality, but would allow the woman, in time, to resume the care of her family mem-ber. Obviously, her circumstances would dictate that this alternative be given closer scrutiny than if she was, for instance, a writer, with a lifestyle that would be much less profoundly affected by the loss of a limb.

But what if one has a patient who is not yet loyally committed to anything? How is the physician to understand such a patient's special needs? I believe we can turn to MacIntyre for help with this question.

LOYALTY, NARRATIVE, AND THE ETHICS OF CARE

Alisdair MacIntyre has claimed that the unity of the individual self consists of the unity of a "narrative embodied in a single life." This view, of course, is close to Royce's view of the self as "a human life lived according to a plan." The notion of a narrative unity, I believe, is especially valuable when questions of loyalty are difficult to answer. Just as the loyalist will always conceive personal loyalty within the context of community membership, the person who has not yet consciously developed the spirit of loyalty will nevertheless view life as a narrative embodied in a social context. MacIntyre writes, "I am not only accountable, I am one who can always ask others for an account, who can put others to the question. I am part of their story, as they are part of mine. The narrative of any one life is part of an interlocking set of narratives" (AV, 218). Even an adolescent boy, who seems to rebel against everything and object to everyone, will tend to define himself in terms of a narrative that includes his conflict with the opposing forces. The youngster will usually be able to give an account of himself that dates back to his earliest memories and will try to relate these memories to his current life by embedding both memories and current life in a coherent narrative. When charged with the care of such an individual, a physician must be attentive to the youngster's story. Even if the patient is no loyalist, the seeds of loyalty are to be discovered only in the patient's narrative.

When discussing care with surrogate decision makers—generally in cases where the patient is comatose, immature, or suffering from an acute thought disorder—the physician should encourage these decision makers to construct a narrative account of the patient's life and to attempt to determine, on the basis of this account, how the patient would feel about the therapeutic options now presented. Such a procedure is entirely consistent with Roycean ethics. As a practical matter, it would often be more effective than querying surrogates directly about the loyalties of their family member or friend.

The process of correlating patients' life stories with their clinical illnesses is only now being investigated in detail (though it has been going on for centuries). Howard Brody has characterized the clinical encounter in terms of the joint construction, by physician and patient, of an illness narrative, couched within the patient's life story. He identifies and explains five important elements of this process: (1) "the patient is fully involved throughout the process"; (2) "the narrative must be meaningful from the patient's point of view"; (3) the details of the narrative must accord with the facts of biomedical science; (4) "the new story ought to promote the healing action that the physician and patient agree ought to be carried out"; and (5) "the new narrative must facilitate either the patient's getting on with his life story or his modifying it as required by the illness" (Brody 1994, 85–87).

The similarities with our Roycean account of the clinical encounter are striking. In both instances, the concern is with interpreting the physical suffering of patients, not merely in terms of a biomedical mechanics but also, and more primarily, in conjunction with an appropriately organized account of the patient's life plan. Only in this context can suffering be understood and remedied. Even more striking is Brody's observation that the attempt to hone this art of joint narrative construction "might represent a sincere attempt on the physician's part to *develop over time into a certain sort of person*—a healing sort of person—for whom the primary focus of attention is outward, toward the experience and suffering of the patient, and not inward, toward the physician's own preconceived agenda" (1994, 88). Like Royce, Brody is acknowledging that, in focusing on medicine's mission of understanding and assisting those who suffer physically, physicians also forge their own personality and realize their own life plan, on a level that transcends merely personal agendas, appealing to higher, community-enhancing ideals.

The writings of MacIntyre and Brody are similar examples of a general and heterogenous development within contemporary moral philosophy—"narrative ethics." Hilde Lindemann Nelson has divided this phenomenon into three categories: (1) where ethicists classify various types of stories in order to use them as paradigms for moral decision making (Jonsen and Toulman, 1988), (2) where literature is studied to enhance one's moral sensibilities, and (3) where persons tell stories in order to make sense, morally speaking, of their lives or situations. As Nelson points out, each of these enterprises is bound to fail if it is not undergirded by some kind of general standard. This standard should consist of an account of the general features of moral life, an account such as we find in the theories of Royce and others. That is, the stories must be anchored by a coherent moral theory.

If one defines narrative ethics as an ethics based solely on one or more of Nelson's three categories or activities, then neither Royce nor MacIntyre could be classified as a proponent of narrative ethics (unless the definition of "story" is expanded to include abstract theorization). On the other hand, if one understands narrative ethics as the enterprise of frequently using narratives—in either of the aforementioned ways—while doing moral philosophy, then Royce is, indeed, a proponent of narrative ethics.[15] In this section we have advocated the utilization of the third variety of narrative ethics—the process of telling stories in order to clarify concrete moral problems. On several other occasions we have appealed to literature to add vividness and nuance to our general theoretical account, thus doing narrative ethics of the second variety. Finally, when we develop an account of the features of certain varieties of clinical problems by appealing to stories such as Ragnar's and Dr. Chester's, we do narrative ethics of the first variety.

Related to the growth of narrative ethics is the proliferation of a clinical "ethics of care." This idea seems to have begun with Gilligan's stimulating (though procedurally flawed) analysis of the moral narratives of children. Based on this analysis, Gilligan divides moral outlooks into two divergent (if not wholly incompatible) outlooks: the ethics of justice, viewed as inherently masculine, and the ethics of care, viewed as feminine. Women, so Gilligan and her disciples believe, view moral life in relational terms. Rather than understanding moral situations in terms of abstract, universal notions such as duty and autonomy, women seek a contextualized account, where responsibilities bear the nuance of multitudinous concrete human relationships. One of the better ways of expressing this nuance is (and always has been) by telling stories—thus, the connection between narrative ethics and the ethics of care.

Gilligan's theory is relevant to our project in this study for several reasons. First, the ethics of care is a fine example of the promising way in which the philosophy of medicine has been enriched by the contributions of original, distinctive thinkers, underscoring Royce's notion that the hallmark of a healthy community of interpretation is the cultivation of individual differences. Second, it contributes to medical phenomenology by introducing the experiences of often neglected members of the greater medical community. We earlier noted that much (though not all) of the outcry about neglecting women in biomedical research is based on disingenuous data shuffling. There is a counterpoint to this insight, however, to be discovered only in the stories of women patients and providers. We will find, should we attend to these stories, that there is more to women's health care than the equitable allocation of funds. Third, the ethics of care is part of the antidote to what is perhaps the greatest failing of applied moral philosophy as a whole: the neglect of the various concrete goods that enhance and inspire moral life. No doubt, the ethics of care has thus far been a little one-sided in characterizing this failure as an inherently masculine folly. Aristotle's account of moral life certainly contained many of the elements—including a focus on virtue rather than the application of moral principles, and an account of the contextualization of virtues—that comprise a contemporary ethics of care. On the other hand, I believe that women, as a whole, and nurses, as the historically female elements of clinical medicine, have indeed been closer and truer than men to the contextual subtleties that characterize an abundant moral life, including a life of loyalty.

Characterizing or criticizing the ethics of care at any length is not within our scope, but a few potential pitfalls of this movement deserve mention, alongside the aforementioned strengths. What troubles me most about the ethics of care, as espoused by one of its leading advocates, Nel Noddings, is neatly expressed in a recent critique of this movement by Hilde Lindemann Nelson:

> Caring advocates' distaste for principles, justification, and reasoned argument can be seen as a kind of ethical postmodernism, in which broad discourse breaks down into fragmented, local conversations. . . . if, in rejecting the commitment to subject our values to the scrutiny of universal reason, we are left with only local and parochial agreement, then we are not going to be able to achieve any real or lasting revision of the social order that systematically bestows greater burdens and fewer benefits on women than on men. (1992, 9)

Nelson here identifies the same problem that we wished to avoid in a narrative ethics—ungroundedness. The failure to support an ethics of care with a reasonable and impartial moral theory (using *reasonableness* and *impartiality* in the limited senses that we developed in the fourth chapter) leads not only to the kind of paralysis in efficacy that Nelson describes, but also diminishes the very notion of "care," since it can no longer be interpreted within the context of a full-bodied, human, moral ideal. How can we strive for the harmonization of ideals or loyalties if the intellectual prerequisites for founding such harmony are thrown out in advance? Noddings's reply to Nelson's criticism (both authors analyze Rorty to explain their positions) is perhaps the most convincing evidence that Nelson is on the mark:

> I do not see why Rorty needs a theory to arrive at the belief that gender equality is wrong. All he needs is the habit of attention and sensitivity . . . and a correspondingly well-developed sense of responsibility (an outcome of habitual motivational displacement). . . . Feeling the pain of those deprived and oppressed leads directly (if we let it) to helping—to standing against gender inequality, for example. Why does he need a theory or master narrative? (Noddings 1992, 16)

How is this sort of subjectivism supposed to get through to an unemployed logger who has recently been abandoned by his fiancée? He too may have cultivated a habit of "motivational displacement," but in his case it is likely to be oriented in a different direction—perhaps toward other depressed, male laborers. Or he may identify with a father who was relentlessly manipulated by a domineering wife. He may be just as motivated as Noddings to "help" by "standing up" against bad people and sinister ideas. But his perceptions will not mesh with Noddings's, and Noddings has no reasonable means of bringing him around. Does she think that merely "standing up" for gender equality—without reasoned argument—is going to move her opponents? It is much more likely to inflame their resistance.

In his essay "Provincialism," while defining the nature of mob spirit, Royce notes two conditions that seem to be embodied in Noddings's thought. First, mob spirit is incited whenever sympathy replaces, rather than complements, thought. Noddings, despite her efforts to exclude forms of sympathy that she finds distasteful, really has no basis for recommending the ethics of care, except that it elicits the sympathies of a select group of listeners. Of course, if the self-legitimization of objects of sympathy is not mediated by some ideal that transcends mere sympathy, then one object is as good as any other. Royce writes that, when sympathies proliferate within a group and reasoned discourse is discouraged or absent, then "the social group may be, and generally is, more stupid than any of its individual members" (RQP, 88). Noddings is not stupid. But many of the groups that traipse about, shouting venomous condemnations and chanting cheap, half-witted slogans, all aimed at "standing up" for some object of sympathy, and that somehow believe that their antipathy will convert others to their simpleminded agenda do, indeed, invite the charge of stupidity. Recall that Royce's moral insight is founded on empathy—where there is insight into the feelings, will, and thoughts of another—not sympathy (based on feelings), and that crucial quality matures only under the tutelage of reason and impartiality.

A second contributor to mob spirit is insularity. Royce distinguishes "wise provincialism" from "false sectionalism" partially on this basis. The social group—whether it be a province, an ethnic group, or some other cultural enclave—that insulates itself from genuine intercourse with diverging social groups is apt, once again, to work itself into a mindless lather over its own narrow-minded agenda. As I have pointed out elsewhere, Royce thinks that the only healthy cultural "diversity" is one that keeps open the channels of communication connecting various groups (1994, 254; 260–261). If Noddings is unwilling to participate in the project of fashioning a means of intercultural discourse—a project that can succeed only if it strives to articulate and cultivate the kind of universal human values that Noddings rejects—then she is, on this point at least, impeding the progress toward a great community.

Perhaps I have misinterpreted Noddings. If so, my qualms about over-localized, under-reasoned versions of the ethics of care still remain as stated. On the one hand, I do not believe that moral life can be totally encapsulated within the notion of "care." With Royce, I prefer "loyalty," for the reasons set out in this study. On the other hand, as I said before, I think there is much to gain by employing the notion of care as a leading idea (one that is adopted because of its fruitfulness, apart from an overwhelming, independent verification of its soundness). There seems to be something elemental about caring, something that is not captured in the notions of duty, goodness, or autonomy. We care even when it is not our duty to care. At times, we care even if we believe that our life would be concretely better if we cared less. And the object of our care is always something more than our own freedom. Caring is part of our collective moral life. It is not everything. But we owe gratitude to thinkers like Noddings and Gilligan for helping us to understand how sorely we have neglected it.

Rights, Rules, and Sticky Situations

In the Pittsburgh Lectures, Royce proclaimed that "if and in so far as you are loyal, your cause it is which defines for you your rights. And your personal rights are sacred in your eyes just because your cause assigns them to you as the treasure you must protect for the sake of the cause." For Royce, the notions of natural and inalienable human rights are incompatible with the philosophy of loyalty and with New Testament scripture. This point needs some elaboration.

A "right" is a claim that someone is justified in making regarding how they ought to be treated by other persons. A "natural human right" is a right that someone has just by virtue of being a human. Since Royce believes that our rights derive from our loyalties, he does not think that there are natural human rights. It is possible to be a human being without being loyal. Therefore, it is possible to be a human being and not have rights.

Does this mean that loyal individuals are not obliged to extend the same basic moral consideration to nonloyal individuals that they would extend to any person who has loyalties? It does not. What it means is that the source of obligation to nonloyal persons does not inhere in those persons. It inheres in the loyalist. In a world without loyalties, the concept of a "right" would be incoherent. Always and everywhere it is loyalty that parents human rights. As soon as someone loyally commits to any cause, that loyalist enters a covenantal relationship with all others who are devoted to the same cause. The loyalist becomes part of a community, with all the rights and obligations that are entailed. In Royce's words, "Your principal right is just the right to serve the cause. And therefore, as loyal person, you know of no conflict between rights and duties. . . . Your rights are your duties to the cause; and your duties are, in the end, your only rights" (RPL I 27).

When the loyal individual subordinates personal loyalties to the highest loyalty—loyalty to the great community—that individual inherits rights that are binding on all morally capable individuals. At the same time, the loyalist becomes obliged to treat all other humans *as if* they were the bearers of natural human rights, since each is a potential member of the great community. This obligation, of course, is incurred by all truly moral individuals.

Are the loyalist's rights inalienable? Presumably not, since loyalty is precarious. On this point Royce cites the parable of the talents (Mat 25:14–30): "The parable of the talents defines, for the loyal, the whole significance that they can attach to the word 'rights.' . . . Your right belongs to you, —yes, but only as the talent to the servant in the parable" (RPL I 26).

The obvious point is that, for Royce, human rights are derivative concepts and not the central concepts of ethics. The correlative points, I believe, are two. First, Royce would hold that the current emphasis on rights is misplaced. Second, Royce would strenuously argue that any account of medical ethics that *begins* with the notion of rights will be inadequate.

These points may be illustrated by looking at "The Patient's Bill of Rights" of the American Hospital Association, which appeared in 1972. This document, which delineates a number of rather obvious patient rights, evidently met with considerable hoopla when it first appeared. The AHA, which provided it for the benefit of patients, apparently to advise them of what they could legitimately demand while confined within the hospital, was praised for infusing the health care environment with a dose of ethics. Nevertheless, I believe that Royce would harbor several reservations with regard to this statement.

First, the tone of the statement is legalistic. It seems to assume that medical practice is fashioned in accordance with the entrepreneurial model. The message is essentially this: Doctors and nurses, along with hospital administrators and other workers in the hospital, are bound to be concerned with their own selfish interests. They will not be, and should not be expected to be, loyal servants of the public interest. But there is only so much that the patient should have to suffer from them. The patient is entitled to certain considerations, here presented.

A second Roycean reservation is that when emphasis is placed on the rights of patients, or, for that matter, on the rights of doctors and nurses, the atmosphere becomes adversarial. Ethics becomes, for the person with the rights, a process of making demands against reluctant authorities. For the person with the correlative duties, it becomes a series of annoying responsibilities. Ethics becomes, as it is often defined, the science of determining just how the claims of one person or group ought to *restrain* the self-interest of another person or group.

Royce would concede that, from the perspective of one at the first level of morality, this account identifies an important function of ethics. But—and this is a third reservation—much of what constitutes ethics is left out. It is through our ethical beliefs that we express our character. It is by our fidelity to these ethical beliefs that we carve our niche in the universe. And it is only through our inclusion in a moral community that any of these beliefs is possible. Ultimately, ethics is better defined apart from the notion of rights, as the science of determining how to harmonize the ideals of one person or group with those of another. Ethics is an affair of cooperation, not confrontation. At times, we have indicated, cooperation will take the form of wholesome competition. But, for Royce, the adversarial approach that is embodied by the tendency to begin with a discussion of human rights ignores the fact that rights are not possible without a preexistent spirit of community. Some harmony is necessary before anyone can legitimately make a demand.

I do not doubt that there is a role for the discussion of patient rights, though I agree with Gaylin that it is not the province of the AHA to determine these rights (Gaylin 1978, 266–267). The fact that we must compose a bill of patient rights is the sad result of the fact that medicine is not invested with the spirit of loyalty. Providers and patients are, indeed, often selfish. We often live as if we were at odds with the rest of humanity. When we are in this mind-set, someone needs to tell us what we cannot get away with. Further, this message needs to come from the health-concerned public, not from the restricted medical community. These rights are not available because they are granted by doctors or hospitals—they emerge out of a mutual covenant. But, if we concede that, in formulating such a message, we have exhausted the subject matter of ethics, or even isolated the heart of ethics, we inflict a mortal wound on one of humanity's finest enterprises.

The same sorts of considerations would apply to a doctrine of ethics based on moral rules or prima facie principles, such as Gert's or Ross's. Gert holds that evil or harm is a more primary concern for ethics than good. Morality derives almost entirely from the obligation to avoid causing evil. The moral rules, which are the centerpiece of Gert's moral philosophy, never demand the preventing of evil or the causing of good, but merely the avoidance of causing evil (Gert [1966] 1988, 74). If one carefully reads the Patient's Bill of Rights, one will find that it, too, requires little else but the avoidance of causing evil. Ross, of course, believes there is a prima facie obligation to bring about good. But he does not ground this obligation in the framework of an eternal community, and, thus, it teeters precariously on the authority of Ross's personal moral sensibilities.

When philosophers hold that rules or prima facie principles are the source of ethics, they relegate virtue to the realm of a strategy. Being virtuous is, at best, a way of living a more satisfying life while habitually meeting the requirements of moral rules or principles. These theories make no requirement to be virtuous.

Part of the clamor for discovering moral rights and principles is no doubt due to the identification of the problem of ethics with the kind of sticky situations that often occur in medical practice. Jonsen marks the inauguration of the era of bioethics with Belding Scribner's introduction of the teflon arteriovenous shunt for hemodialysis. He gives two reasons for this association: (1) it caught media attention, and (2) it was an early case of the problem of allocating scarce medical resources (Jonsen 1990, 17–18). Both of these reasons highlight the role of bioethics as an instrument of resolving a special brand of problems that arise within the context of medical practice. I call these the "sticky situations," and they have several characteristics. First, they are rare. Part of the reason they cause such a stir is that each of them falls far outside the normal scope of everyday medical practice. Second, they are controversial. No consensus forms around how these problems should be handled. Third, they involve matters of great importance. Whether or not I point out the string hanging from my patient's nose is a problem that arises only rarely, and I know of no consensus that can guide me on how I should address it. But, because of its triviality, the string-hanging-from-the-nose affair is no sticky situation.

Dealing with sticky situations is important—important enough that we have addressed some of them in this essay. But, to Royce and all virtue ethicists, these situations can never occupy anything but the periphery of ethics. Even so-called "applied ethics" should be primarily the enterprise of describing a certain realm of loyalty. In order to deal with the truly sticky situations, one must first have a general moral outlook.

The new clinical casuistry, championed by Jonsen and Siegler, often begins with sticky situations and develops certain moral principles by attending to paradigmatic cases. Little or no reference is made to moral principles that exist apart from analogous cases.[16] There is much to commend this approach. First, it recognizes the truth that philosophy always begins with a problem situation. Second, it eschews remote moralization in favor of guidelines that are both relevant and practical.

Nevertheless, I believe Royce would have reservations about this brand of casuistry. The casuist does not seem to recognize sufficiently that the most important practical problems are those of a very general nature. Who am I? Why should I go on living? What is a good life? Because the casuist neglects these problems, he does not discover just how important their solutions can be for the approach to sticky situations.

Royce speaks not only to the casuist but also to those who are overly concerned with rights or moral rules and principles when he criticizes those who hold that

> the moral law is or ought to be a collection of precepts, an exhaustive collection—one adapted to all possible situations, and of such a nature that, if you are confronted by a difficult situation, you have only to look into your moral code to find somewhat clearly set down just what it is that you ought to do in this case. (RPL II 1–2)

Later he adds:

> No, whoever seeks simplicity and clearness as to his duty must seek it in the form of simplicity and dutifulness of spirit, not in the form of a memorized set of maxims, suitable to all individual cases that may arise. (RPL II 4–5)

Most of what separates morally good physicians from morally reprehensible ones occurs outside the framework of sticky situations. Good

physicians are those who exhibit virtue in every aspect of their professional lives, not just on the rare occasion when confronted with a particularly difficult case. Of foremost importance is that physicians develop
the spirit of loyalty. This requirement is not only their highest ethical duty
but the key to living the good life as a physician.

We have dealt with some of the ways in which an ethic of loyalty will
have bearings on the grand tradition in medicine, examining some of
medicine's central moral features and challenges and exploring the inter-
face between Royce's thought and a variety of other, contemporary philosophical orientations toward the same subject matter. In the final chapter,
I will briefly summarize some ways in which a medical ethics of loyalty
might be interpreted by individual physicians.

8

❖

The Loyal Physician

Samuel Shackelford did not speak often. When queried about his illness, his cursory replies came in a voice so quiet and tentative that one had to strain to hear them. His deference was almost excruciating. Suggestions and advice from his third-year-medical-student caregiver were accepted as if they issued from the lips of God or Zeus. He was a black man, perhaps only in his late fifties, but with a withered exterior and gray hair that made him look more like seventy. The manner in which he cherished his pouch of chewing tobacco produced the same effect, as though he had discovered the futility of worldly pursuits and found peace in something simple. His apparent antiquity made his standard conversation—"Yes sir" "No sir"—all the more awkward for his still-pimpled medical student.

Mr. Shackelford was my first patient on the first day of my general surgery floor service in my third year of medical school. He was admitted to receive a sympathectomy in order to relieve chronic lower extremity pain, which was related to peripheral vascular disease, or PVD. The PVD was caused by his tobacco use, an activity that was especially reviled by my caffeine-addicted chief surgery resident, Dr. Pinhart. From his elevated perch, Dr. Pinhart identified tobacco use as one of the signature characteristics of the common "dirtball"—he was horrified to learn of my own snuff-dipping habit and forbade me to indulge it while I was on his service. Shackelford, however, offered me a bit of his chaw, and, despite my guilt about undermining one of the goals of medicine, I took it. In this transaction, our mutual affection was cemented.

I scrubbed in with Dr. Pinhart on Mr. Shackelford's operation. As per the norm, I was queried about the operation, then treated to Pinhart's exposition of its intricacies. He informed me of several possible complications but reassured me that Mr. Shackelford should have no problems— after all, "you can't kill a dirtball," as Dr. Pinhart often said. (I wondered if this was a proclamation of his own immortality.)

After the operation, Shackelford remained comatose for several days. I remember sleeping in and making it to the hospital barely in time for 0700 rounds. When it came time for me to report to Dr. Pinhart on Mr. Shackelford, I confessed, with mortified seriousness, that I had not yet visited him that morning. Dr. Pinhart smiled: "Well, I can tell you he's stable." My relief was short-lived. As I looked upon Mr. Shackelford's dead body, my embarrassment was swallowed up by a sinking heart. Meanwhile, my companions had a good laugh.

In retrospect, Samuel Shackelford was a great teacher. Through him, I learned very early about the harshness of medicine. I learned that "dirt-balls" can be more honorable than their medical saviors. Most importantly, he taught me about quiet human dignity. The contrast between his humility and Dr. Pinhart's arrogance was striking. In his slow, unassuming manner, Mr. Shackelford invited me to become a better person, to emulate his wise simplicity, and to honor the lofty standard that he assumed would be the norm among medical professionals. Sadly, he received nothing in return, save a few moments of relief from the loneliness that infests hospital wards, a loneliness foreshadowing a death that went virtually unnoticed, except for some brief hilarity and the lingering memories of a young medical student.

Josiah Royce was impressed by the manner in which moral lessons could be imparted by actions.[1] As Mr. Shackelford shows us, one need not preach—or even have much to say—in order to cultivate loyalty. Leadership by example is much more striking. The loyal physician is, first of all, one who has heeded the call to such leadership. This call echoes in the words of Albert Schweitzer, who was a minister before he studied medicine:

> What seemed most senseless to my friends was that I wanted to go to Africa as a physician, not a missionary. This meant at thirty years of age a long, difficult period of training. I had no doubt myself that the project would require an exceptional effort. . . . I wanted to be a doctor so I could serve without hav-

ing to talk. . . . My calling as theological teacher and preacher
was certainly a source of satisfaction to me. This new calling
appeared to me, however, to be a matter of putting the religion
of love to work rather than of talking about it. (Schweitzer
1965, 163)

The physician, by virtue of his esteemed social role, as well as his
helpful presence during periods of sickness and vulnerability, has a unique
opportunity to inspire loyalty in others. Often, he fails. Sometimes it is
the patient who must be the moral teacher—as in the case of Mr. Shackelford. But part of the task of medicine is to work at lifting the burden of
moral or spiritual emptiness, which contributes as much to physical suffering and destitution as any microbe or autoimmune catastrophe.

If medicine, with its tradition and its practitioners, is to succeed in
this task, it must first attend to its own spiritual lethargy. Recall the third
criterion for revising a tradition discussed in chapter 6—the practical criterion. When we apply it, we ask whether or not a tradition can sustain
us. We have already assaulted the grand tradition several times from the
vantage point of this criterion. We have commented on the sterility of
rules and rights. We have pointed out the inadequacy of dogmatic formulations in the face of the current skepticism and relativism. And we
have argued that only an ethics of loyalty is true to the passion that ignites
the human spirit—the search for identity and meaning. On this basis we
have already used the practical criterion to justify a modification of the
grand tradition in the direction of a philosophy of loyalty. Nevertheless,
much practical work remains. Most of it is work that cannot be done by
philosophers alone.

If Royce is correct, genuine loyalty is our collective destiny. Each of
us shares in the future of the great community. Royce, the philosopher,
helps us think about this destiny, but his guidelines are general. They provide us with a strategy and leave the tactics to us. In the long run, each
person must refine the individual art of loyalty. Each of us must construct
and adorn our cause into something he or she can cherish, so that it stirs
true devotion rather than mere intellectual assent. An abstract philosophy
is not enough to sustain us. We are creatures of passion. We need more.

For Royce, this "more" is largely a matter of religion. Many clinicians,
no doubt, share his religious proclivity. The power of religious imagery is

immense and needs no introduction. The Roycean endorsement of religious liberties is designed, in part, to unleash this power on behalf of the great community. If Royce is correct, it is only through religious devotion and divine grace that we can fulfill our destiny. I do not wish to challenge this opinion. (In fact, I agree with it.)

But there are other images—available to both religious and nonreligious individuals—that are also potentially useful. William F. May has claimed that a central task of ethics is to provide "corrective vision" by investigating the manner in which we view the world and by making suggestions about how it should be improved (May 1983, 13–14).[2] One way of going about this task is to develop and investigate various metaphors. These metaphors are tools that we use to flesh out our images of the morally good life. While very general metaphors and ideals are the domain of philosophy or ethics,[3] more specific metaphors will be applicable only locally. An orthopedist, for instance, may be inspired by conceiving his mission in analogy to that of a master sculptor. An internist may see herself as a sleuth. Each of the more specific metaphors will appeal to certain personalities more than others. They will also apply to certain specialties better than others. Each carefully crafted metaphor becomes a sort of template for a unique loyal life—the projection of a moral narrative. In fact, as we fill in the details, we find there are an infinite variety of possibilities for embodying loyalty in a life story, with a corresponding infinitude of possible metaphors.

To apply the practical criterion to the grand tradition in medicine is to work with metaphors, both broad and specific, and see how they fit our clinical lives. It is an affair of the imagination, wherein we tell our professional stories on a personal level. Our view of the clinical virtues will fall in line with these stories.

Each of us must undertake this task, to a degree, on our own. Nevertheless we feed on one another's efforts, recognizing the bonds of community.[4] It is in this spirit that I now proceed.

In this final chapter, I will provide a brief portrait of how the revised tradition might work in the lives of loyal physicians. Specifically, I will point the reader in the direction of a virtue ethics for medicine, based on loyalty, by discussing the virtue of honesty. I will also discuss a metaphor that I have found valuable in the practice of emergency medicine—the image of the warrior.

Honesty

Virtues, we are told, are character traits or ingrained habits. Through our habitual ways of acting and thinking, we establish our identity, which is to say, we define ourselves through our virtues and vices. Royce wrote that "Your cause is just your own self writ large" (RPL I, 23). This statement is designed to convey the comprehensiveness of loyalty. For Royce, it is the virtue of loyalty that encompasses all the others. It is through our own peculiar form of loyalty—the comprehensive virtue—that we express ourselves to the world.

Our cause allows us to define habits as good or bad—as virtues or vices. No virtue is comprehensible apart from the cause to which we are loyal. Thus, to act courageously is to serve our cause well under dangerous conditions. Courage, along with all the other virtues, is a subspecies of loyalty. If we commit some daring act in order to prove we are superior, with no appeal to a cause, then we are rash. In this case, our behavior is the expression of vice. Loyalty is the characteristic to which we appeal when we judge all other characteristics. If we are energetic, we count this as a virtue if it helps us serve our cause. If, on the other hand, an excess of energy causes us to be distracted from some task we have loyally undertaken, then it is a vice.

One of the most important virtues for Royce and Cabot is honesty. Cabot thought is was so important that he wrote a book about it (Cabot 1938). Royce discussed it at length in RPL. His comments provide a valuable summary of the relation between loyalty and the subordinate virtues.

He begins by noting that, though honesty is an important virtue, loyalty is occasionally best served by telling a lie. He illustrates with the example of a prisoner who is interrogated about the plans or whereabouts of his unit. How should such an individual express loyalty to loyalty? Royce tells us that the prisoner should make no secret of his devotion to his unit and his country. By his obvious loyalty, he forewarns his captors about the result of any interrogation. It is as if he says, "My obligation to them is higher than my obligation to speak truthfully to you." They should expect him to lie. When he misrepresents the whereabouts of his unit, he honestly serves his cause. He cultivates the spirit of loyalty, not only by being faithful to his fellow soldiers, but by giving his captors a dose of his dignity and honor.

Royce does not comment about the option of simply not speaking. Perhaps this would generally be the most acceptable option for the genuinely loyal prisoner. However, it is not difficult to envision scenarios where the prisoner would serve loyalty better by lying. One of the Knights Hospitalers—Adrien de la Riviére—provides a courageous example of such a contingency. When tortured by Mustapha during the siege of Malta, Riviére cried out that Mustapha should attack the Castile, since it was the weakest point in the Knights' defenses. Just the opposite was, in fact, the case, and Mustapha lost hundreds of men finding this out. In return, he had Riviére beaten to death (Bradford 1972, 149). With his lie, and his willing acceptance of the certain torture and death that followed it, Riviére aided his cause heroically.

But Royce continues that it is *almost never* necessary to lie or to mislead others. The physician who makes a habit of smugly ending every patient interview with exaggerated characterizations about the brightness of the prognosis is a case in point. This practice can lead to a loss of credibility:

> The physician who systematically misleads his patients as to their true condition, loses his power to say the really comforting and inspiring word when his patients are beset by false anxieties. (Royce RPL II, 26)

Royce continues later:

> On the whole, lies told to keep sick people in good spirits fail of their purpose. One of our heaviest dreads, when we are weak and suffering is often this, that we justly fear lest our best friends will now deceive us for what they take to be our good. One of the first things to do if you have to help a nervous sufferer is to win his confidence. And in the long run you cannot win his confidence unless you deserve it. (RPL II, 39)

Cabot rightly associates the physician's impulse to lie with a failure to educate his patients. Cabot notes that physicians often feel compelled by the expectations of patients to come up with a firm diagnosis. He points out that this expectation is often unreasonable and that it is predicated on ignorance (Cabot 1938, 135–136). Patients often harbor the false belief that a good physician ought to be able to arrive at a fixed, certain diagnosis quickly and efficiently. When a doctor caves in to this assumption, he perpetuates this ignorance and may harm his patient. An example is the too common scenario where a patient presents in the early stages of acute appendicitis. Often there is no accurate way that the physician can diagnose the illness at this stage. Yet there are instances where physicians have told these patients they are suffering from "gas" or "indigestion" rather than honestly informing them that the etiology of their pain is not apparent and that, though it might be something transient, they should return if they experience continuing pain or worsening. The patients who are falsely reassured are apt to delay treatment when they worsen.

We have already seen that educating patients is a primary task of the loyal physician, an idea Cabot enthusiastically reinforces, tying it in with the imperative to be honest:

> The speed of our development towards entire truthfulness about the diagnosis of disease will depend largely on how hard doctors work to educate their patients. Thus far the medical profession has left the medical education of the public mostly to nurses, social workers, and the medical columnists of the daily press. But the doctor himself can do this teaching better if he will take the trouble, and if he does not share the ancient illusion that "a little knowledge is a dangerous thing." . . . We can lessen the danger only by increasing the knowledge. As the doctor educates his patients he will descend from the pedestal of exclusive expertness on which he has allowed tradition to keep him. Patients will share some of his knowledge and apply it to their own uses. That is the result which anyone who cares for health must hope for. Unless people learn to take care of themselves far better than they now do, general health will not substantially increase. Medicine and surgery will never accomplish this. Public health work can do something. But the practicing physician can do more than anyone else if he will systematically educate his patients. (1938, 148–149)

In these words, Cabot expresses nicely the spirit of his departed teacher.[5]

In denouncing "the pedestal of exclusive expertness," Cabot touches on another virtue, closely related to honesty, and certainly more neglected. That virtue is humility. Humility stands somewhere between the polar vices of arrogance and self-deprecation. Of the traditional seven deadly sins, arrogance and greed seem to be the most treacherous obstacles for contemporary medicine. We have already spoken of greed. Our characterization of Dr. Pinhart is an introduction to arrogance. As many have noted, science and its child medicine have become contemporary idols. There is a growing tendency to view technology as a universal panacea. For the sick, this tendency is manifested in the common belief that life can be easy, once again, if only one succeeds in finding the right therapist. Medical professionals can themselves be hypnotized by this belief. As the high priests of the new secular faith, they are greatly esteemed and are apt to become inordinately self-impressed.

The problem here, of course, is that life is rarely easy, clinical medicine is highly imperfect and greatly limited in scope, and clinicians, for their part, are as prone to human frailties as any other group of individuals. Further, the incompatibility between arrogance and genuine loyalty should be apparent. If I am a loyalist, I am, first of all, a fallibilist. I must always be cognizant of the possibility that I have worked out the details of my loyalties incorrectly. There is no room for arrogant dogma. Second, as a loyalist I am committed to achieving social harmony—something that is not likely to occur if I habitually approach the views and practices of others with self-righteous disdain. This is not to say that I should not stand up for I believe is right. Not to do so would be to embody the opposite vice, self-deprecation, and shortchange my cause. But I should carry out my defense in a spirit of humility that recognizes the manifold intricacies, and the unknown destiny, of my beloved great community, always mindful of my small and fallible part in its creation.

THE MILITARY VIRTUES

The most important image discussed by William May is that of the "covenantor," one who views one's professional life as the expression of a sacred covenant with patients. May's image of the covenantor is similar to the one we have discovered, and largely approved, in the work of Pellegrino and Thomasma. May observes, in *The Physician's Covenant*, the existence of a central image for this book does not altogether dismiss the other images. They have a place. . . . Correspondingly, the covenantal image accommodates in principle for the healer's activities; it warrants them all. But alone the image does not throw important features of the healer's task into sufficient relief. The images of parent, fighter, technician, and teacher still clarify. (May 1983, 23)

Royce believed that loyalty is enhanced by augmenting it with concrete images. Though the ideals of hero, self-denying self and rebel were treated as competitors with loyalty, Royce sought also to strengthen the image of loyalty by assimilating the better elements of these alternatives. Recall, additionally, how he identified three species of loyalty by looking at family structures.

Regarding May's noncovenantal images, we have already discussed aspects of the technician and the teacher. We treated the image of parent— as well as that of spouse (or friend) and sibling—when we discussed the manner in which the physician-patient relation reflects familial strains of loyalty. The image of the loyal healer as a fighter, however, has not been considered here at any length.

Before we talk about the warrior, I would like to stress, once again, the huge multiplicity of images that could be employed by individual practitioners in order to vivify their notions of loyalty. May and Royce have hit on only a few of the possibilities. Kleinman serves up some more, in the form of his medical narratives. In what follows, I will not be claiming that all physicians are warriors, or that this metaphor is appropriate to all clinical situations or human personalities.[6] Instead of the warrior, I could have written of the physician as sleuth, an image that is portrayed brilliantly by A. J. Cronin in *The Citadel* ([1937] 1965) and which I find very attractive. But, at this point in time, I find the warrior more intriguing. What follows is largely personal.

Military virtues, I believe, do not always get the attention they deserve, perhaps because they are so prone to excess and are, therefore, associated closely with vices. But if it is hard to identify, to image, the representative or typical examples of a class of virtues, that is all the more reason why they should be studied carefully.

We took a military view of things at a couple of prior stages in this essay. In chapter 3 we talked about Rommel's natural loyalty, and in chapter 4 we talked about the connection between loyalty and the war spirit. Several reservations were voiced about military models. We mentioned the disastrous effects of violence on the cultivation of loyalty, as well as concerns about mob spirit and the confusion of sympathy with empathy. Regarding Rommel, we noted that his natural loyalty was not yet genuine loyalty, since he seemed to lack a conception of the great community.

Nevertheless, we also noted how the military can be a natural breeding ground for loyalty. Further, the flaws we found in Rommel's general philosophical views did not keep us from appreciating the unusual dignity and integrity with which he lived. I believe, in fact, that there are other lessons we can learn from individuals such as Rommel. As an emergency physician, my practice has been enriched by studying military strategies. I have enjoyed the martial arts not only for the physical stimulation but also as a source of practical guidance and inspiration.

Let us begin by looking once more at the life of Field Marshall Erwin Rommel. We know he was a legendary figure during World War II. That he exemplified characteristics such as courage, honesty, and common sense has rarely been questioned, even by his critics. These are timeless virtues, important to warriors and healers alike, spanning the chasm between Rommel's battlefield and our own hospital emergency departments. Certainly we can benefit from emulating them. But I have something different in mind.

Biographer David Fraser, himself a former British general, has identified three keys to Rommel's genius (1993, 5–7). First, Fraser notes: "The master of the battlefield has always relished the challenges of combat. . . . Battle is his element." There is ample evidence that Rommel felt deep pain over the brutalities of war. His reflections on war were colored by a spirit of mercy. He was always chivalrous toward the enemy and appalled by those who were not. He was enraged by reports of excesses towards civilians. Nevertheless, there is no doubt that, in the throes of battle, Rommel, deeply competent and energetic, experienced a kind of inner harmony and satisfaction, characteristic of the master whose skills are put to the test.[7] Rommel was a warrior. Combat was his business, at which he excelled. He plied his trade with the cool efficiency of a professional. In this regard, Fraser cites the experience of a captured British officer:

A British officer who drove in error into the Sidi Muftah area, not knowing that 150th Brigade had been overrun, found himself suddenly a prisoner, standing under guard next to a car in which Rommel sat, directing the battle of the Cauldron, an armoured radio car on either side of his own, handing scraps of paper with his orders scribbled on them first to left then to right, reading the battle and very obviously directing it entirely personally, utterly calm, utterly in control, as it seemed utterly confident. The contrast with what the captive had seen of British command was sharp indeed. (328)

Rommel was more than just competent and sanguine under fire. He was relentless. In the first world war he had been a lieutenant in charge of four companies in the Alps. After a frigid night march, then the occupation of Jevszek, and a successful frontal assault on the stoutly defended Mount Cragnoza, Rommel and his Alpine corps did not rest. Instead, they initiated several skirmishes and fought their way to the threshold of Mount Matajur, a key strategic location held by the Italians. He then received an order to withdraw. But, correctly surmising that the order was based on misinformation, Rommel once again moved ahead. His forces quickly took Mount Matajur. In fifty-two hours of unremitting activity, Rommel and a few hundred men took over nine thousand prisoners. In an earlier battle, at Mount Cosna, Rommel went five days, saturated in blood from a wounded arm, without pausing long enough to remove his boots or change his bandage. He reported that "all were in fine spirits!" Three days later he led a successful six-day assault on Mount Cosna, capturing and holding the objective. At the finish of the battle, he was running a high fever and babbling, according to his own recollections, "the most idiotic stuff" (Fraser 1993, 59–61). In France during the initial Western offensive of World War II, Rommel once again eschewed recuperation. After leading the 7th Panzer Division through several French strongholds and over the Meuse, Rommel was ordered to rest his troops at least two days. Instead, he persuaded the authorities that they were in pursuit and must apply the old Prussian maxim—"Pursuit should be to the last breath of man and beast" (Fraser 1993, 181).

Rommel, we see, was a synthesis of virtues that many hold to be antagonistic. He was boundlessly energetic while imparting an aura of composure. He was fervent, yet calm. He fought with a will of iron—cool, capable, unrelenting. Such an attitude is expressed by the Japanese term *bushidamashi*, translated as "warrior spirit."

The second virtue identified by Fraser is more elusive. He designates it with the term "understanding," but far more is expressed here than what we generally attribute to this term. Understanding of the type referred to by Fraser has only a tenuous relation to theoretical knowledge. Knowledge of theory is necessary. But more important is the kind of knowledge gained from experience and repetition, the kind of knowledge that dwells within the muscles and reflex arcs, not the head. Fraser writes:

> But understanding and knowledge of war, at the sort of pitch where it distinguishes the great battlefield commander, in some way surpasses the cerebral. It becomes a sixth sense, an instinct, a gut reaction beyond such phenomena (equally essential but more easily describable) as the ability to judge a situation and an opportunity shrewdly and instantly. . . . It lies in that which men called Erwin Rommel's '*Fingerspitzengefühl*' his almost animal response to the dangers, the chances, the currents of battle.

The concept of *haragi*, from Japanese martial arts, parallels the notion of *Fingerspitzengefühl*.[8] The former has been translated as "intuitive thought," or, more descriptively, as "a state of mind that eliminates the harshness of reality." Royce, despite his unathletic nature, was quite aware of this quality, of how it is fostered by physical training, of the part it plays in loyal living. In RQP, Royce quotes a mountain climber, Philip Stanley Abbot, who describes a dangerous descent in the Selkirks:

> I had been feeling lifeless all that day, and we had already had nine hours of work. But the memory of that next hour is one of the keenest and most unmixed pleasures I have carried away,— letting one's self go where the way was clear, trusting to heels alone, but keeping the ice-axe ready for the least slip,— twisting to and fro to dodge the crevasses, planning and carrying out at the same instant,— creeping across the snowbridges like snails, and going down the plain slopes almost by leaps,— alive to the

fingertips,— is a sensation one can't communicate by words, but you need not try to convince me that it isn't primary. (RQP, 279–280)

Experiences of this variety are apt to occur whenever someone highly trained in an intricate skill is acting with profound mastery. The clumsy mechanisms by which we usually integrate thoughts and acts are shed, and, briefly, the master performs flawlessly, in a state of thoughtlessness that is often described in mystical terms.

Fingerspitzengefühl is related to warrior spirit. The warrior who thoroughly internalizes the skills and strategies of combat is able to function in a subconceptual state, as if by instinct (and probably to a degree actually by instinct), so that he experiences battle more as a harmonious discharge of energy than as a situation where he is confronted by a fulminating chaos of threats, counterthreats, and hard decisions. He exists in a state of *mushin*—"no thought, no ego"—and becomes impervious to horrors such as the fear of death.[9]

One who exhibits *Fingerspitzengefühl* does more than just react to stimuli. He is an initiator as well. And, whether he acts or reacts, his techniques are, in Fraser's words, "applied with instancy." This is the third, and culminating, virtue of Rommel's battlefield persona. Rommel had a peculiar ability to enter a theater of operation with its established rhythms, drawn from a thousand strategists, and transform it immediately and violently into his own personal hunting grounds. He would initiate engagements without warning and without apparent deliberation. Should he take time to deliberate, the enemy would have time to anticipate his deliberations. But there was no time, no hesitation. Further, once he was successful in an engagement, he would almost always move immediately to another, taking full and methodical advantage of any disruption of the enemy's composure or morale. In so doing, Rommel would impose his own inner workings on the pace of battle. He would employ, once again in the words of the Japanese, *ichi no heioshi no heiho*—the strategy of the rhythm of one. That is, he operated by subjecting the chaos of the battlefield to the control of a singular will.

We should note that the "one" in the "rhythm of one" is ultimately, according to Zen Buddhism, not a single person, such as Rommel, but is the inexpressible unity revealed in enlightenment. This fits in more closely with the manner in which Royce interprets the perceived unity of social endeavors. He would hold that we ought to strive, in every activity, to manifest the greater, metaphysical unity of the beloved or great community, rather than our own will understood as a merely personal possession. For Royce, this is possible even in conflict.

As we have remarked, the image of the healer as a warrior is nothing new. May calls attention to the prevalence of military terminology in the hospital and also to that setting's military-style hierarchy of command (1983, 64–66). The emergency department, especially, is like the battlefield. It is a place of blood and dying, of confusion and high emotion. It is a place where tranquility does not come naturally. Somehow, the masterly emergency physician, like the masterly field marshall, must learn not only to survive but to thrive under these conditions. This is accomplished, ultimately, when the practitioner is able to focus on two targets: the enemy, to be dispatched; the prize, to be won.

We have talked about both the enemy and the prize at length. The former is suffering and death. The latter is health and, at a higher level, the cultivation and harmonization of loyalty. May has characterized medicine's enemy as death:

> Modern medicine has tended to interpret itself not only through the prism of war but through the medium of its modern practice, that is, unlimited, unconditional war. Before the twentieth century, the West, by and large, subscribed to the notion of a just war. A just war, no matter how just its cause, had to offer some prospect of victory. Further, a just war required a careful limitation on the means used to fight. But in the twentieth century, the democracies, as well as the totalitarian states, waged total, unconditional war with the commitment of all means, extraordinary as well as ordinary, to the victory. Just so, hospitals and the physician-fighter wage unconditional battle against death. (1983, 66)

He then correctly goes on to identify a complication—often it is suffering, not death, that provokes our desire for medical intervention (1983, 68). We have already claimed that medicine's *summum malum* is suffering. My point is that the warrior spirit in medicine requires a special, adversarial attitude toward this enemy. Doctors fight suffering.

Likewise, the dedication of the physician to the health and well being of his patients should be as focused and intense as Rommel's devotion to the honor of Germany or the samurai's devotion to his lord. The physician can learn from the single-mindedness of these models. When he walks into the clinic or hospital, his concern for family affairs, for the upcoming political elections, or for the fate of his favorite football team must be suspended. He is there for a purpose. To that purpose he must be true.

Royce's reflections about a speaking engagement are illustrative:

> A newspaper once asked me to contribute to a so-called symposium whose problem was to be this: What characteristics will the ideal man of the future possess? As I only knew about the ideal future man this, that when he comes, he will, as in him lies, adequately attend to his own business, I felt unable to contribute anything original to the proposed discussion. (RQP, 154–155)

His point is that the day-to-day business of being loyal will, for the most part, consist of single-minded devotion to doing one's job and doing it well, and further, that the characteristic virtues that contribute to success will depend upon the nature of the job and the nature of the individual, which are rather unspecifiable in advance.

Besides intensity and focus, there is another aspect of warrior spirit that warrants close attention by physicians. We remarked that Rommel relished combat. I believe that the physician who excels at medicine will relish his clinical challenges as well. Royce follows Aristotle, who held that, though virtue rather than pleasure is the good, virtuous activity will generally be pleasurable. We are creatures who define ourselves in terms of our characteristic activities. When we excel in these activities, we are pleased.

The second special warrior virtue noted by Fraser is *Fingerspitzengefühl*, or what we called "intuitive thought." *Fingerspitzengefühl*, Fraser would tell us, cannot be taught directly. It is the insight gained through years of experience and dedication, molded together with our special talents. Nevertheless, our mentors can point us in the direction of this virtue. The tools of one who wants to train for *Fingerspitzengefühl* are repetition and harsh conditions.

When we perform the same tasks over and over, we condition ourselves to perform them without thought. The karate student who practices a front kick fifty times a day will, in the period of a few years, be able to perform a flawless front kick effortlessly. Likewise, the medical student who practices a one-hand surgical tie every evening before bed will eventually be able to perform the tie unconsciously. The same sort of conditioning occurs with more complicated skills. After we have assessed several thousand patients with acute abdominal pain, we will internalize certain aspects of our procedure so thoroughly that we will undertake them without thought. The experienced surgeon does not need to be reminded that patients with inflamed peritonea will move slowly and deliberately. The surgeon picks up on this automatically. Doctors learn to go with their "gut feeling" because it is a synthesis of insights that have incredible cumulative power.

No matter how much we practice, no matter how accomplished we seem to be in the classroom, we often seem to wilt when we hit the front line. How many times have we seen a highly touted quarterback fall apart in his debut? How often does the medical school ace need to be rescued by an experienced nurse when he falters before his first code blue? There is, unfortunately, no substitute for training under fire. Once again, the Japanese have a term—*chugyo*—for training in harsh conditions. The idea is that if you can spar in bitter cold and rain, or sweltering heat, you are more likely to perform creditably under the pressures of genuine combat. The traditional grind of medical and surgical residents is backed by a similar insight—if you learn to do it without sleep, you will be able to do it all the better when you are rested. The "mega-code" in ACLS (Advanced Cardiac Life Support) training is another analog to *chugyo*. In this, the final stage of testing for ACLS credentials, students are hammered from every angle as they try to resuscitate a manikin. The condition of the manikin will change more quickly and more dramatically than any real patient they are likely to encounter. The time they have to make a decision will be substantially less than with real patients. Most clinicians will tell you that the mega code is more stressful than handling a genuine code blue. If so, all the better. No one wants his or her life to hang on the decisions of a doctor who has never known pressure, who might be trembling instead of acting.

Iserson has noted that we are apt to make good moral decisions when we have rehearsed similar decisions in the past (Iserson, et. al 1986, 36). His point is that we have to train for moral virtues in the same manner that we train for other clinical virtues. The success of these enterprises will depend, to a degree, on whether our training includes adequate repetition and exposure to harsh conditions. When young Dr. Mary Phillips is beset with a difficult moral decision, or has an unsatisfactory social interaction with a patient, she should reflect on this experience in the same manner used when reflecting on a difficult diagnostic challenge. Our young physician must constantly question herself about her moral ideals and how they are expressed in her professional behavior. Perhaps, through this reflection, Dr. Phillips will develop some useful moral rules of thumb—maxims about promoting loyalty that are similar to those of the casuists. Even more importantly, she will infuse herself with her cause. If she thinks about it every day, it will become a part of her. Regard for her cause will come to be expressed automatically, without thought.

We have noted that the physician should put aside all nonprofessional concerns when arriving at the clinic or hospital. Yet one of the central messages of this essay is that professional concerns must be integrated with our whole life. The key to balancing these two requirements is in the aforementioned process of repetitive prior deliberation. The loyal physician has deliberated about the requirements of professional life at enough length to become comfortable with the relation between medical and personal ideals. A (sometimes provisional) harmony between these aspects of personality is achieved in advance, before donning the stethoscope.

Through deliberation, repetition, and strenuous training we can internalize our ideals. When we succeed at this task, we are no longer fickle or prone to debilitating moral indecisiveness. We approach every situation with the confidence that we are firm in our commitments. We are in a state of mind that mitigates the harshness of reality.

The third of the triad of warrior virtues described by Fraser is the most difficult to understand, but perhaps the most important. I favor the Japanese term for this virtue—*ichi no heioshi no heiho*, or "the strategy of the rhythm of one." The chaos of illness is analogous to the chaos of battle. Both can be overwhelming and destructive. The competent physician, like any other competent leader, is one who can bring the force of his or her personality—and, ultimately, the unifying spirit of a cause—to bear on the present chaos. This physician is one who can render the discord into order. We have commented on Rommel's ability to assert himself nonverbally. Gandhi pioneered the same quality in India:

> Throughout life, Gandhi explored new fields of communication. Sometimes he would go to a huge mass meeting, but instead of delivering a speech he would sit cross-legged and sway and say nothing and then he would smile and touch his palms together in the Hindu greeting and the crowd would kneel and weep. He had communicated. (Fischer 1954, 75)

Ichi no heioshi no heiho is a form of nonverbal exchange. It is a way of taking charge instantly. Three things occur when a master exhibits this virtue, but it is of fundamental importance, especially in combat, that these three elements be "applied with instancy." There is no mechanism, only a single act.

First, the master takes in a situation instantaneously, without thought. Using the Japanese metaphor, the master has a "mind like the moon." For the warrior, this means that he takes in everything at once and therefore quickly perceives the weaknesses in his opponent's defense. For the physician, this means tuning into the mood and qualities of the patient's thoughts. The physician enters the patient's inner life, or, perhaps more accurately, the patient is allowed to enter the physician's inner life. Without saying a word, the physician becomes privy to the patient's suffering. Each of us has had the experience of "receiving strong signals" from another person. When we have a mind like the moon, we are especially receptive to these signals.

The second feature of the rhythm of one is an instantaneous exchange of energy. In combat, this exchange may be violent. The seventeenth-century samurai warrior Miyamoto Musashi wrote:

> Among the rhythms used to strike an opponent, there is what is called a single beat. Finding a position where you can reach the

opponent, realizing when the opponent has not yet determined what to do, you strike directly, as fast as possible, without moving your body or fixing your attention. The stroke with which you strike an opponent before he has thought of whether to pull back, parry, or strike is called the single beat. (Musashi 1994, 24)

In medicine, the exchange of energy between the physician and patient is not violent. It is of the nature of an infusion. The patient is weak and tired—life has soured. The patient may have lost the resolve to weather any further storms and is pessimistic. The physician responds to this privation of spirit by thrusting comfort and enthusiasm. Like the blow of the samurai, the physician's offering is relayed in an instant, taming the ravages of illness.

But in this case the most common weapons are a smile and a look of confidence. The move is effective only because the physician also takes on the patient's suffering, not just sympathetically, but empathetically. Therefore, the physician's smile is the patient's as well. It is part of their burgeoning mutual endeavor, of their shared community.[10]

Finally, there is an effect. For the warrior, the effect is the defeat of the enemy. For the physician, it is not only initiating the defeat of the enemies, suffering and death, but also rekindling a spirit of loyalty and optimism in the patient. To impart such a benefit quickly is not easy. It requires experience and patience. The physician must cultivate the twin abilities of apprehending and nourishing the aspirations or problems of another.

The rhythm of one is a worthy ideal for the loyal physician. Here there is a single movement, which is neither of the physician nor the patient alone. It is the rhythm of their two lives, joined by empathy and compassion into a mutual, constructive clinical endeavor. Ephemeral plans and lost missions come into harmony with an eternal ideal.

Mother Teresa and the Missionaries of Charity complete each day's mass with the following words:

Let me preach you without preaching, not by words but by my example, by the catching force, the sympathetic influence of what I do, the evident fullness of the love my heart bears to you. Amen.

These words reverberate with the rhythm of one cause. In her gentleness, Mother Teresa appropriates and transforms the warrior's virtue for the healer's art.

Perhaps the most difficult task for the student of Royce is to reconcile his many abstractions with his pragmatist's call for practical relevance. Yet this reconciliation is a central aspect of Royce's philosophy. For Royce, as for Mother Teresa, the distant perfection provides animating grace. Life is a series of local struggles. The glimpse of the eternal is a clarion, calling the loyalist to an ultimate victory. Animated by loyalty, the physician finds in each clinical encounter an opportunity for fulfillment and service—service to patients, service to the community, and service to something greater still, something beyond our grasp, yet present, palpable, indelible.

Notes

Bibliography

Index

Notes

Introduction

1. cf. Jonsen 1990

2. cf. Cotton 1954

3. Insofar as we succeed in our task, we will have offered evidence that they are commensurable.

4. Emphasis is MacIntyre's.

5. Royce's most cogent criticisms of Hegel are contained in his unpublished lectures (Oppenheim cites "The Spirit of the Community," in volume 91 of the Harvard University Archives Royce Collection). Published accounts include his article "Two Philosophers of the Paradoxical" and *The Spirit of Modern Philosophy*.

6. Hocking (1912, 158) has aptly applied the term "volitional idealism" to Royce's voluntaristic metaphysics. Hocking's critique of Royce's voluntarism would almost certainly be accepted by MacIntyre.

7. Compare MacIntyre's comments about Sidgwick on p. 28 versus p. 78 of *Three Rival Versions of Moral Enquiry*.

8. It is interesting to note that, according to Royce, the decline of teleology has not resulted in a historically unprecedented state of affairs. Royce's unpublished lectures on the history of ethics begin, unlike *After Virtue*, with an examination of moral traditions that emerged centuries before Greece. Royce notes that primitive morality was not teleological: "Notice that here is little or no thought of any higher end that is immediately served by obedience to the supposed supernatural will, or any higher end of this will itself" (LHE, Lecture 1, 21–22).

9. To explain this difference in outlook, it would probably be useful to examine the degree to which it is influenced by the thinkers' respective metaphysical differences regarding the debate between voluntarism and determinism. Royce strongly aligns himself with the former position. MacIntyre has showed sympathy for the latter, which, Royce would say, is not surprising given MacIntyre's realism. Royce's comment that realism is inherently conservative (WI I, 73–75) might also lend some insight into the fact that MacIntyre tends to be somewhat more conservative than Royce. These considerations, if developed, would lead us too far afield of our objectives in this essay.

Chapter 1

1. This is not to say that modern bioethics only offers the ED physician advice to

practice according to the standard of care. Such is certainly not the case. Rather, I am commenting on a trend in the way ED physicians view their profession. E. E. Smith comments on the existence of fifteen hundred practice guidelines, aimed at delineating a standard of care (1993, 1196). See also *ACEP News*, May 1994, for a discussion of the importance of meeting the standard of care. I will have more to say on this matter at a later juncture.

2. Robert Williams, past president of ACEP, in the lecture entitled "Key Public Policy Issues for Emergency Medicine: The Next Five Years," delivered at the 1993 ACEP Scientific Assembly, comments on how the Clinton health plan would have exacerbated this contradiction.

3. For example, Dolan et al. (1993) asked twenty-five low-risk patients with recent upper GI bleeding whether they wanted diagnostic endoscopy, upper GI radiography, or no routine testing. Diagnostic endoscopy is the most accurate of the three for detecting a bleeding source, but is also the most expensive, the most uncomfortable, and the most risky. In most low-risk patients the results of diagnostic endoscopy will have no bearing on treatment, since the various causes of minor upper GI bleeding are each treated with the same sorts of medical regimes. Nevertheless, 92 percent of patients chose endoscopy. Twenty-two physicians were queried on the same issue, and only 55 percent chose endoscopy. See Baraff et al. (1994) for a case where patients opted for less invasive procedures and less risk.

4. Nuland notes that the historical confusion is probably based on the fact that some of the Hippocratic physicians called themselves Asclepiads (7). It is interesting that Aristotle (who was a youth during the twilight of Hippocrates' career and who later spoke of "the great Hippocrates") was the son of an Asclepian physician. Certainly Aristotle's understanding of medicine is far more in line with the Hippocratic physicians than with the Asclepians.

5. It could be argued that altruism, as a motive *distinct* from that of living a happy life, could have no place within Greek ethics. For Aristotle, any virtue, including kindliness or altruism, is understood simultaneously as an end in itself and as part of a happy life. The tension between altruism and egoism did not exist for the Greeks as it does in the modern mind. We will return to this issue later.

6. In the CPC, the clinical record is correlated with pathological findings, generally obtained at autopsy. The autopsy findings provide information about the accuracy of diagnosis, and the effect of therapeutic interventions. Of course, this information provides the basis of discussions about how things could have been managed more effectively.

7. The CPC was, no doubt, quite a blow to the "gentlemanly model" of medical ethics that was espoused by Percival in 1803. Pellegrino and Thomasma note that "Percival's ethics of 1803 provided all the moral precepts and even some of the words for the AMA's first code of ethics (1993, 34)."

8. MacIntyre responds to this mistake by discussing how traditions are "historically extended, socially embodied" arguments (AV 222).

9. There are, of course, other causes of impersonalism in medicine. Excessive specialization and the reliance on advanced technology come immediately to mind.

10. We will discuss COBRA—the "Consolidated Omnibus Reconciliation Act"—at a later juncture. The intention of this legislation was to prevent patient dumping. Though relatively successful at achieving this important end, it has also caused hardship for patients and physicians alike by transforming the process of patient transfer into an exercise in bureaucracy.

11. Interestingly, in a recent summit with representatives from the three "primary care" specialties and emergency medicine, President Clinton and his advisors were totally unaware of this pervasive but ridiculous legislation and had to ask to have it read to them.

12. Clouser and Gert (1990) have attacked "principlism," but the alternative that Gert puts forth in *The Moral Rules* would be nearly as susceptible as principlism to MacIntyre's complaints about theoretical patchwork.

Chapter 2

1. Lectures in the History of Ethics were delivered early in Royce's career, before he was established as a prominent American philospher. Though Royce's thought evolved considerably after LHE, his ideas about the conditions for intellectual and political revolutions were not so much altered as enriched, so that the passages quoted from LHE are, in my opinion, congruent with his later position.

2. In my doctoral dissertation, *The Loyal Physician: An Essay Applying the Ethics of Josiah Royce to the Practice of Medicine* (1995, 81–91), I treat Royce's theory of the development of personal identity in more detail than I will here. In that work, I compare Royce's theory to that of a current psychologist—Roy Baumeister—showing that Royce's views are echoed by the latter thinker (though Baumeister was not directly influenced by Royce). This section of the dissertation is recommended to those who think of Royce's theory of psychological development as antiquated.

3. Royce's ideas on docility are similar to what we see later in the philosophy of John Dewey, especially in *Human Nature and Conduct*.

4. Baumeister (1986, 18) identifies "continuity" and "differentiation" as the two "defining criteria" of identity. These are achieved, to a substantial degree, through imitation and opposition, respectively.

5. Daniel N. Stern points out that imitation goes two ways. Parents imitate the early smiles, monosyllables, and other important early behaviors of their infants. In so doing, they act as a kind of mirror for the infants, who learn that they are persons like their parents. It is interesting that Stern cites Baldwin, whose descriptions of imitation had a profound influence on Royce (Stern 1985, 8; 127; 137–138).

6. Likewise, it is not possible to will, in the wider sense, the possession or knowledge of an object if one has no experience of such an object. This thesis is an aspect of Royce's notion of the relation between internal and external meanings (WI). Knowledge,

for Royce, is a distinctly purposive activity. The internal meaning of our ideas is the expression of their purposeful nature. The external meaning of our ideas—essentially, the external object to which these ideas are directed—can never be something of which we have no prior experience or conception. Royce's account of voluntary behavior in OP is best viewed as a specialized example of the more general account of the expression of purpose from WI.

7. Recall Royce's opinion from LHE that revolutions are inherently conservative. This thesis ties in with his notions about novel ideals.

8. Royce cites James as a proponent of this view (OP, 289).

9. The "middle period" for Royce's ethics is 1896–1911 (Oppenheim 1993, 61–84).

10. Oppenheim observes that the middle Royce "aimed to balance true individualism and loyalty and to simplify the conceptions of good and duty," whereas by 1915 "he had clearly identified the 'three leading ethical ideas' and harmonized them with the idea of the loyal Self." He goes on to suggest that this is a dimension of Royce's growth during his final year (Oppenheim 1993, 16 n.14). No doubt, Royce's notions of duty and goodness flowered during his final years, but it is also clear that the middle Royce saw loyalty as a comprehensive ideal, synthesizing these other central ethical ideas. The discussion of rights and duties in RPL (7–8) is one example of this vision. This passage also illustrates how the middle Royce did, indeed, subordinate the concept of duty to those of individualism and loyalty. In the later Royce, the concept of duty is more fundamental— both as an ethical concept and as a psychological insight—than it is in the middle Royce. It will be incumbent upon us to take account of this development in our subsequent discussion.

11. Note the contrast between Royce and thinkers such as Kant and Butler, who maintain that native human reason, or a faculty of conscience, is adequate to the task of constructing a moral outlook.

12. With Roy Baumeister, Royce would insist on three general reasons why a personality ideal—i.e., an authoritative metacriterion of identity—is important: (1) it helps us to make choices, insofar as it provides us with a system of values, goals, and priorities; (2) it helps us to establish and maintain interpersonal relationships, insofar as it is constituted by socially recognized roles; and (3) it endows us with a sense of resolve, insofar as it is constituted by a devotion to specific ideals (Baumeister 1986, 19). These are, of course, the general psychological functions of a personal identity. As we shall see, Royce goes further, claiming that without such a metacriterion—without a coherent personal identity—human life is wretched and meaningless.

13. Royce's hero should not be confused with Emerson's.

14. MacIntyre writes that "morality and social structure are in fact one and the same in heroic society (AV, 123)." Of course, the society that created Marcus Welby is not the heroic society of ancient Greece. MacIntyre states the obvious when he says that

"Nobody now can be a Hector or a Gisli (AV, 126)." Further, it is quite possible to interpret Marcus Welby as something other than a hero. He might be viewed as a loyalist. My point, though, is that those who sought to emulate Welby generally looked upon his character as a kind of heroic personality. Welby is analogous, in the ways we have described, to Hector or Achilles.

15. Royce also refers to this ideal as "the saint." "Self-denying self," as we will see, expresses more fully the range of manifestations of this basic concept of personality.

16. It is not "we" collectively who are identical to the metaphysical will. Schopenhauer does not believe in a collective whole. Instead, he maintains that each individual is an appearance of the "whole, undivided . . . being in itself." (Schopenhauer 1958 II, 590–591).

17. Søren Kierkegaard also attends to the notion of a self-denying-self. Kierkegaard, with Schopenhauer, describes both aesthetic and mystical forms of self-denial. Kierkegaard sides with Royce, however, in rejecting the ideal of the self-denying-self. Similarities between Royce and Kierkegaard are striking, at times, but should come as no surprise. Both are influenced by Hegel. Each objects to Hegel on the grounds that he ignores or denigrates the subjective element of human experience, and that he overestimates the capabilities of a single human intellect, regarding especially the breadth of historical and conceptual insights, while at the same time underestimating the significance of the individual's unique life. Kierkegaard ultimately has less use than Royce for concepts, since, unlike Royce, he recaptures some of the scope he stripped from Hegel through a highly particularized, nonconceptual, absolute relationship with the absolute. In contrast, Royce's human individual remains forever fallible, with never more than a highly imperfect glimpse at the absolute, and must carve out his niche with whatever tools, conceptual or volitional, he can find.

18. In later years, Albert Camus emerged as another giant of this variety. Camus rejects suicide, because, once he understands the absurd, he recognizes how the meaninglessness of life elevates the individual to prominence (Camus, 1955).

19. This is not to say that he sought the eradication of valuation in the face of the historical character of values. Rather, he sought ever newer expressions of value, recognizing that values soon become old and stale—impediments to the creative force out of which they emanate.

20. Interestingly, Nietzsche recognizes this incompatibility. This insight leads to an attempt at rejecting the self. Nietzsche's philosopher is characterized as "a storm pregnant with new lightnings (1966, 230)," lacking the structure of a self; he is seized by a will to power that is more primordial, more creative, more unpredictable than one could express in the rubric of selfhood. If the philosopher is by necessity the possessor of values (in the sense of ideals), he is nevertheless the medium for a force that has no ideal. The only value that consistently comes out in the philosophy of Nietzsche is the affirmation of this force. Such an affirmation, once it is expressed as an ideal, becomes divorced from

its own primordial energy. Thus, insofar as it expresses the structure of selfhood, it is an artifact, energy blocking energy. Nietzsche, so viewed, preaches not a philosophy of self-affirmation, but merely a philosophy of affirmation.

21. When the priest laments that Rieux has not been converted, Rieux's response reflects the same spirit of unity, as well as the tension Rieux experiences regarding his unlikely alliance: "'What does it matter? What I hate is death and disease, as you well know. And whether you wish it or not, we're allies, facing them and fighting them together.' Rieux was still holding Paneloux's hand. 'So you see'—but he refrained from meeting the priest's eyes—'God Himself can't part us now'" (1948, 197).

Chapter 3

1. See PC 162–163, 169, 175. Here Royce writes of the "hell of the irrevocable" experienced by those who commit treason.

2. Though I refer to this definition as "preliminary," it is important to note that Royce never overturned it. Ten years after PL, it appears again in PC (83). Royce's subsequent definitions were considered complementary, highlighting other important aspects of loyalty. The preliminary definition served well—and still does—as a way to introduce loyalty to a new audience.

3. We have said that the cause is something that exists apart from the existence of the loyalist. This point does not seem to apply to causes that arise in the formation of certain small, exclusive communities, such as a community of two lovers. One could counter that loyal lovers are dedicated to *eros,* which exists apart from their particular union. This may be true much of the time. It seems to me, however, that most lovers are dedicated to *their love,* which is not the same as being devoted to love in general. Nevertheless, their love is something that transcends their combined personal characteristics.

4. Later in his career, Royce came to prefer talk about communities over talk of causes, though the notion of a basic equivalency between causes and the interests of communities was never abandoned (PC, 83, 174–175).

5. A problem with George Fletcher's book *Loyalty* is that he never clearly makes the distinction between true loyalty and authoritarian loyalty. Royce himself is, on rare occasions, guilty of the same oversight and, in fact, makes no terminological distinction between these two forms of loyalty. Nevertheless, Royce clearly regards authoritarian loyalty as a degenerate form of loyalty (PL 55) or, at times, not loyalty at all (RPL III, 44–46). Though both forms occur in Fletcher's examples, he more frequently represents loyalties as authoritarian, and this bias affects his conclusions. The reader should be careful to note that "true loyalty," as we here define it, covers both natural and genuine loyalties, as defined by Royce (our discussion of these will follow). Fletcher misrepresents Royce's notion of genuine loyalty, but this difficulty is only obliquely related to the fact that he fails to distinguish between true and authoritarian loyalty.

6. If the individual is not unique, he is not an individual. The uniqueness of each individual consists of the fact that he/she is an irreplaceable object of God's attention. I know of no way of extricating Royce's notions of individuality and freedom from his theology. For the purposes of this book, I will be content to say that Royce thinks that the individual's choice of a cause is made freely. Kucklick (1972) has excellent discussions of Royce's accounts of individuality (43–48; 109–110) and freedom (115).

7. Advisors later prudently persuaded Rommel to delete the word *political* from this sentence.

8. cf Fraser's account of Rommel's response to a request from South African soldiers that black prisoners be segregated from white. Rommel turned down the request "flatly, saying that the blacks were South African soldiers, had fought alongside whites, worn the same uniform and were all captives together (338)." Remarkably, Rommel once suggested to Hitler that he promote a Jew to an important post, apparently oblivious to the fact that Hitler did, indeed, hate Jews (132).

9. Royce used the terms *First, Second,* and *Third* in PC. I prefer not to use these terms, because I think they might lead to confusion with the Peircian concepts of Firstness, Secondness, and Thirdness. Oppenheim (1994, 816) also uses the term *principal* as the first term in the triad, and this use apparently follows Royce's use of the term in "Spirit of the Community" (an unpublished work that has been examined by Oppenheim but not by me).

10. There is a passage in SGE where Royce claims that, once thoroughly habituated, so they function "as by a mere instinct," virtues are no longer matters of "active moral goodness" (SGE 111). This idea reflects his insistence that morality and struggle are unseverable. I believe, however, that the mature Royce would have reservations about this statement, and I agree that the thoroughly habituated virtue, when attained by struggle, will always be significantly unlike an "instinct," and will, in fact, possess a moral blessedness unrivaled by the as-yet-to-be-internalized virtues (PC 132–133).

11. Hocking and Marcel have pointed out that, for Royce, there is no direct intersubjective communication. Thus, in Royce's view (Hocking and Marcel do not agree), one becomes acquainted with the thoughts of another only through the medium of physical signs. This issue is discussed by Daniel S. Robinson (1968, 72–74).

12. To my knowledge, Royce never explicitly confirms his agreement with Peirce that a person is a sign.

13. The letter to Elizabeth Randolph exhibits an aspect of Royce's humanitarianism that should not be missed. Royce did not endorse the "bleeding heart" variety of philanthropy that seeks to establish, with a single stroke, lasting happiness and contentment for all. He sought, instead, to help the world by constituting his own life as a moral example. In RPL, Royce states: "To try and deal out simple happiness to mankind at large is like persistently plying them with wine. One in so far makes them at best stupid,— perhaps vicious" (III, 29).

14. I am indebted to Frank Oppenheim for pointing out this latter form of degenerate loyalty, though the term *parasitic* is my addition.

15. That Gandhi never read Royce, and never used the term "great community," is beside the point. There is no doubting that Gandhi was committed to a harmonious community of all humanity.

16. In 1921, Gandhi wrote that the caste system was "essential." By 1932, he called it "debilitating." See Fischer, pp. 111–112.

17. Interestingly, in 1946 he declared that no marriage would be performed at the Sevagram Ashram unless one of the parties was an untouchable. The emancipation of untouchables remained a central issue for Gandhi after his epic fast.

18. Those doubting that Royce was a fallibilist should recall that, throughout his career, Royce's argument from error formed the intellectual foundation for his absolute idealism. Royce is thoroughly aware that this argument hangs on the truth of an unproven premise—that we err. This leaves open the possibility that there is no error and that philosophical theories (such as his own idealism) are neither true (in any strong sense) nor false nor even erroneous, but either simply meaningless or valid from some highly particularized perspective. For Royce, even the principles of logic are objects of interpretation, to be revised in accordance with human purposes (Oppenheim 1987, 50). Most importantly for our project, Royce stressed the fallibility of all moral ideals (PL 169–170) and the constant need to revise one's moral ideal in a spirit of humility (Oppenheim 1993, 139–140). (My thanks to John Stuhr for alerting me to the need for this clarification.)

19. The "Beloved Community" is the great community, graced by the Holy Spirit.

20. For Royce, this form of naturalism would render his moral idealism a meaningless call in the dark. In his view, it was dispatched by the arguments of *The Religious Aspect of Philosophy*, establishing the existence of an absolute being who insured an eternal moral order.

21. See *Death Be Not Proud* (Gunther 1949, 221) for a layman's perception of how God shares in human suffering.

22. The idea of a program of mandatory service of the underprivileged (generally two years) for all physicians has occasionally surfaced. This notion makes good sense, fitting, as I believe it does, with notions of social justice. Such a program would not, however, be a truly atoning enterprise, unless it were invested with a spirit of loyalty. Since loyal service is always willing—and not coerced—I doubt that such a mandatory program would fit the bill.

23. I became fully aware of this emphasis through the work of Frank Oppenheim (1993, 162–163; 170–171). References to ECE are based on his research.

24. Royce's disavowal of ultraconservative political formulations is evidence that he would not have held that traditions should be maintained without alteration unless overwhelming arguments to the contrary are presented.

Chapter 4

1. Royce distinguishes between loyalty as an ethical need and a psychological need early in PL and indicates that he will consider it first as a psychological need (PL, 21–22).

2. See my discussion of the mob spirit in "Royce, Community and Ethnicity (1994, 253–54;265)."

3. I will not take up the tedious subject of the extent to which the individual's readiness for sacrifice is a genuine turning away from selfishness. There are thinkers who insist that every act of service or sacrifice is really an attempt to further one's own interests. This view becomes somewhat credible when one considers that, once one has taken on the well-being of another person as one's own concern, the well-being of that person becomes a part of one's own well-being. It is this kind of insight that causes Royce to abandon the distinction between egoism and altruism altogether. My only concern in demarcating the levels of moral life is that we acknowledge a shift in orientation. At the first level the moral agent is not directly or consciously concerned with the well-being of other persons; at the second level the moral agent is so concerned about others that willingness to sacrifice more individualistic concerns on their behalf comes easily. It would be hard, in my opinion, for proponents of universal egoism to explain why an atheist would risk life and limb to save a drowning child—these and many other similar, common events defy the egoist paradigm.

4. When I describe the moral insight as an act of mediation, I am adding content to Royce's primary account of this insight, contained in RAP. I believe that my description coheres with Royce's mature ethical theory, represented in PC and his Extension Course in Ethics. Most of my version of Royce's moral insight, however, is contained in chapter 6 of RAP.

5. Fuss correctly points out that two other principles are included in Royce's characterization of the moral attitude in RUL—(1) respect for persons and (2) harmony (147–151). It is my view that these two principles are corollaries of reasonableness and impartiality. In RAP Royce shows at some length how the principle of harmony is a byproduct of the moral insight.

6. Of course, this image reappears in Aristotle's account of the intellectual virtues and their primacy.

7. "The Moral Philosopher and the Moral Life" includes the following footnote: "All of this is set forth with great freshness and force in the work of my colleague, Professor Josiah Royce" (James [1967] 1977, 628). In the note, James refers specifically to ideas about the place of a divine thinker in ethics. But, as Clendenning notes (1985, 139–40), James's initial response to RAP as a whole was very favorable.

8. Royce does not discuss the valuations of nonhuman sentient beings in his discussion of the moral insight.

9. This imperative is categorical in the sense that it applies to all actual moral agents. Royce would not hold that it was a categorical imperative in the strictly Kantian sense that it necessarily applies to all rational beings. It is logically conceivable that there is a rational being who does not will unity. Royce supports the current consensus that a categorical imperative grounded solely in the concept of rationality does not exist.

10. The tediousness of such a world devoid of striving or conflict is one reason for celebrating the fact that we will never, from the standpoint of finiteness, achieve an end to moral inquiry. James was sporadically quite aware of the psychological need to have the satisfaction of our desires impeded, but he misses the boat altogether in this essay.

11. Here Royce's ethics runs parallel to Peirce's epistemology. Both are predicated on the validity of the quest to mediate between ostensibly divergent sets of data.

12. In fact, Royce's "moral insight" is, in RAP, a stepping stone towards his more profound "religious insight" (436–474). This connection is something that Royce worked out for the ramainder of his life, refining both insights significantly. Royce's aforementioned notions of interpretation, community, atonement, and spirit were all developed, for the most part, after RAP, and all contributed to his mature doctrine of loyalty. We have already (as I previously noted) enriched RAP's account of the moral insight by accomodating it to Royce's later notion of interpretation, and our account of loyalty in the preceding chapter incorporates manifold elements of thought from the later Royce. For a chronological development of Royce's moral theory, I recommend Fuss (1965). The best comprehensive account of Royce's mature ethics is contained in Oppenheim's book on this subject (1993).

13. Royce points out in LHE that the Platonic ideal differed in certain ways from the post-Homeric Greek popular ideal of Plato's day.

14. In a manner befitting Royce, Elie Wiesel wrote, "God made man because he loves stories" (1966). We have already briefly discussed the relation between Royce's individual, loyal, life plans and MacInyre's moral narratives. With an infinity of possible details, there are bound to be as many concrete instances of loyalty—and therefore as many distinct instantiated moral ideals—as there are loyalists. Royce, anticipating some of the insights of our modern "narrative ethics," gloried in such diversity. This attitude, once again, undescores his reservations about trying to express loyalty in terms of neat formulas or definitions but does not detract from his message that there is unity in diversity—that all genuine loyalties come together in the hope of the great community.

15. And, ultimately, all sentient beings. But we will confine our discussion to humans.

16. The difference between Schopenhauer and Royce, once again, is that Royce believes such a state can never be achieved from a human frame of reference and, further, that any achievement of moral perfection must be the result of struggle. The great community viewed from the standpoint of the infinite is a lost cause for flesh-and-blood human beings. The apparent paradox of a loyalty that seeks its own obsolescence arises only because we counterpose the infinite to the finite.

17. Recall, in *Symposium*, that Diotima shows Socrates that, if the gods possess the beautiful and the good, then Love cannot be a god, since Love seeks the beautiful and the good but does not possess them. In essence, we have made the same observation with regard to Loyalty. Diotima holds that the spirit of Love is an envoy or interpreter, plying between heaven and earth. Loyalty has the same function in the religious life described by Royce, and, thus, the metaphysical description of the great community has an important religious function.

18. We can fashion this point in terms of the usual division of actions into intentions and results. Intentions are, for Royce, more important than results. The problem with this division is that it is not very sharp. Intentions are themselves frequently results. When we aim to cultivate loyalty, we try to bring about certain intentions as a result of our actions.

19. Royce, as we have previously pointed out, does not claim that this moral insight is the permanent possession of morally praiseworthy individuals. He claims only that such individuals will be able to transform this fleeting insight into a new ideal and should achieve, incrementally, an increasing sense of moral unity as they pursue it.

20. Even mathematics is, for Royce, a moral endeavor. The mathematician is one who seeks to describe certain universal, abstract relations between numbers, forms, and operations. The discovery of these relations is his cause. This cause, like any other, is the object of human will, of desire. Like any other ideal, the ideal of the mathematician is valuable because of its relation to human fulfillment. It must be evaluated alongside other competing and complementary ideals. Further, mathematical relations are not merely valuable for individual mathematicians, who find fulfillment in study, but also as an aspect of that total unity that is the aim of the will to interpret.

21. In this paragraph we have viewed loyalty to loyalty through the lens of one of Royce's three leading ethical ideas—duty. Throughout most of this study we have, thus far, given more priority to the other leading ideas—goodness and autonomy. We have argued, with Royce, that loyalty is the ideal of a morally good life. We have also spent a great deal of time in discussing how the ideal of loyalty integrates the principle of autonomy with the notion of a good life.

22. Royce's complete argument for this position, of course, is contained in WI.

Chapter 5

1. Ultimately, we will want to classify it as a *triad*, rather than a dyad, but I am ahead of myself on this point.

2. Classicists may have observed that we employ an Aristotelian approach here. In essence, we began by identifying the material cause of the clinical dyad—two human persons—and then queried about its efficient, final, and formal causes.

3. Richard Zaner points out that the patient has already interpreted his experiences before he appears before the physician (Zaner 1988, 173). The patient's self-interpretation may be very simple, as in a groan or other expression of pain (recall our discussion

of how "ouch" is an interpretation), or very complex, as when a patient presents with a definite opinion about his diagnosis and how his illness should be managed.

4. Perhaps the reader is already uneasy about the term *dyad,* since the aims of the "dyadic" community are clearly being mediated by whatever social factors account for the physician's "special training and skills." If so—good!

5. Interestingly, Royce states in WAR that loyalty must always involve relations between more than two persons (34), contradicting two of his examples in PL (11,25). There are two ways that we can explain this contradiction: (1) the examples of loyal lovers and loyal friends in PL are a mistake, i.e., Royce does not really think that one can be loyal to a dyadic community; or (2) the statement in WAR concerns genuine loyalties, where the loyalty to a given community always involves a built-in appeal to loyalty to greater, more inclusive communities, whereas the example of the loyalty between lovers is given as an example of natural loyalty. Support for the first of these interpretations comes from Royce's comments later in PL, where he refers back to the example of friendship as an example of a cause "which unites several friends into some unity of friendly life," possibly implying that friendship between only two parties is not a locus of loyalty, and his comment in WAR that "the normal family is not a pair, but at least a triad, a group of three persons: Father, Mother, Child (37)," apparently implying that the stability achieved in families cannot be obtained through the union of lovers in a childless marriage. Nevertheless, I support the second interpretation, pointing to the fact that, in the same paragraph in which he claims that loyalty always involves more than dyadic communities, Royce also claims that dyadic relations between friends can be stable when they appeal to higher relations, or "because love takes the form of true loyalty." In either case, it is clear that loyalty to a dyadic community is possible only if the ideal of this community expresses more than any member of the community can conceive or pursue as an individual, and that such expansiveness of the ideal is ultimately possible only because of relations, explicit or latent, between the dyad and polyadic social groups (thus situating the dyad of persons within a triad of interpreters).

6. The clinical dyad, viewed on the entrepreneurial model, is not even a community in the limited sense discussed above.

7. Actually, as we will see, it may be more advantageous to look at the physician as a mediator of the relationship between medical science and the patient. Though I will not stress it here, it is noteworthy that most triadic relations between principal, interpreter, and interpretant can be rearranged conceptually. We have already noted that any interpretant may serve as a principal. In many triadic relations, each of the three elements serve, in part, as an interpreter, though the degree of involvement as the interpreter is usually asymmetrical. Recall Zaner's description of the intertwining interpretations that characterize the clinical encounter.

8. Proponents of the entrepreneurial model virtually always recognize the same need. Their manner of fulfilling it, however, is vitiated by their basic view of morality, as we shall see.

9. Hocking and Marcel disagree, as Robinson points out in his lucid analysis of these thinkers (Robinson 1968, 73).

10. By "theorization" I refer to a process similar to what Peirce calls "abduction."

11. This is the familiar law of Laplace. For cylinders with one radius of approximately infinity, it becomes T=PR. That is why capillaries have thin walls and the aorta has a thick one—the pressures are similar, but the radii, and consequently the wall tensions, differ greatly.

12. For those who need a reminder, interpretation is a process by which the principal is explained, translated, or otherwise directed by an interpreter toward an interpretant. The interpreter thus *mediates* the relation between principal and interpretant.

13. By "community of interpretation," Royce means any community that is defined by ideals that emerge and are realized largely through the triadic process of interpretation. Royce's most general account of the community of interpretation seems to be contained within PC (315–317). In WAR, he describes four types of community of interpretation: (1) the judicial community, (2) the banker's community, (3) the community of insurance, and (4) the agent's community (WAR, 56). This list is far from exhaustive. There is probably some credence in classifying the scientific community as a kind of agent's community.

14. Also, persons who are health care workers who present to clinicians with an illness suspend their roles as health care workers, and, for the moment, are members of the lay public. The surgical nurse, for instance, does not scrub in on his own appendectomy.

15. One of the important aims for future research should be to determine certain general situations in which standard clinical measures do not apply. These situations are engendered not only by individual variations, such as we find in Mr. Storaasli's case, but by cultural and ethnic variations as well.

16. I am a little uncomfortable associating the parent-child relation with the leading idea of duty. I think this move is vulnerable to the feminist criticism that "parent" is here understood more as "father" than as "mother." The fact is, however, that Royce seems to envision parenting more explicitly in terms of motherhood than of fatherhood (PC 128). Perhaps Royce's notions of motherhood are colored by his own masculinity. And perhaps among the leading ideas of ethics a fourth should be added—that favored notion of many feminists, caring. Indeed, the importance of caring permeates much of Royce's discussion of the moral life—not merely in regard to the family but also in his treatments of "the cult of the dead" (HGC, 93–95) and love as a source of religious insight (SRI, 37–75). It would be wrong to view Royce as an opponent of caring, though it is true that he would eschew an ethics based entirely on caring just as thoroughly as he eschews ethics based solely on autonomy, goodness, or duty. We will discuss the "ethics of care" in chapter 7.

17. Thanks to Frank Oppenheim, whose influence is manifest in this section (as well as several others), but who should not be blamed for its inadequacies.

18. Veatch classifies activity models of medical ethics as "professional physician ethics."

19. Veatch calls it "impartiality," but what he means by this term is better captured by the term *equality*. In any case, *impartiality* in Veatch's hands is something radically different from what it is in Royce's hands.

20. If Veatch is correct here, i.e., if the obligations at the second and third levels derive from the first level, then the edifice of his medical ethics is susceptible to the devastating criticisms that can be brought against his basic social contract. I suspect, however, there are reasons supporting some of these obligations that are not related to his social contract.

21. At times, Veatch seems to claim that physicians do not have a special insight into health or the alleviation of suffering (and also that professional ethicists will not have a special insight into what is right). He loses me here. If this is so, why do we sanction these practices in the first place? And why did he write his book?

22. Veatch might use this point to answer our first criticism. He could deny the legitimacy of the present "contract" that he thinks exists between society and the medical profession, since it was not made from the moral point of view.

23. The term "sectarian" has unfortunately acquired some derogatory underpinnings. By a "sect" I will mean simply a group of people forming a distinct unit within a larger group. I know of no other term that captures this meaning as well. The common ascription of qualities such as narrowmindedness, dogmatism, or insularity should not be made. As we will soon discuss, it is quite possible for a sect to bear these negative features. But it is also possible for sects to bear the characteristics Royce assigns to his "wise provincialism."

24. Royce's response to Balfour's skepticism in RAP is similar to this response to Veatch and Engelhardt.

Chapter 6

1. The inclusiveness of the greater medical community is, once again, the reason why Jonsen can speak of the effect of the "old ethics" on patient attitudes (1990, 10). That is also why it is only natural that the public should have a say in reforming the tradition—through political or other social measures.

2. It should not be inferred that Royce rejected the "Christian" version of altruism. Many Christians have supported a version of altruism that corresponds with the one Royce advocates (Ashley and O'Rourke 1989, 14).

3. The similarity between Plato's and Royce's theory on this point should be obvious.

4. There are, of course, forms of "enlightened" egoism that hold we are happier when we pursue ends that are traditionally associated with altruism. These theories approach the moral insight. Egoists of this variety have bridged the gap between egoism

and altruism. What should be noted is that it serves no purpose to call them egoists. Just insofar as they genuinely pursue altruistic motives they are altruists. The ideal of such enlightened egoists is close to the ideal of the loyalist. The enlightened altruist, for analogous reasons, is also close to the loyalist.

5. Royce indicates in RPL that one of the principles of "the Art of Loyalty" is "In case of the appearance of conflict, look beneath the superficial conflict to find if possible the deeper common loyalty, and act in the light of that common loyalty" (2: 50). Oppenheim's discussion of the motion of "fittingness" in Royce's mature art of loyalty is illuminating on this point (1993, 137, 140–142).

6. The source here is *U.S. News and World Report* (October 30, 1995, p. 106), which cites the Medical Group Management Association. The data for reports such as MGMA's is obtained by survey and may, in fact, underestimate the real gap between generalists and procedure-oriented specialists such as radiologists (Larson 1996).

7. Recall Royce's principle of autonomy.

8. I will not tackle the difficult task of constructing a theory about what constitutes coercion. The kind of independence I describe here is what Gerald Dworkin has called "procedural independence," which is freedom from coercive influence. He distinguishes it from "substantive independence," which he does not define, but which he seems to regard as the freedom from any kind of influence (coercive or uncoercive) from other people. Dworkin writes that he is unable to conceive of a way in which loyal or compassionate actions can be regarded as independent in the substantive sense, since they are actions that "are to some extent determined by the needs and predicaments of others." He continues: "Again, any notion of commitment (to a lover, a goal, a group) seems to be a denial of substantive independence and hence of autonomy. There seems to be no way of conceptualizing substantive independence that avoids this classification (Dworkin 1977, 26)." Royce would counter that the loyal individual is one who has freely aligned his own interests with those of a community, so that his personal needs are no longer distinguishable from those of the community. He would hold that the independence of the loyalist is the only genuine form of substantive independence. It would be impossible, I believe, for Dworkin to give us an example of a single action or decision substantially independent in his sense.

9. See Robert Nozick, *Anarchy, State and Utopia* (1974, 28–30).

10. Cassell wrote, in 1977, "I believe that the function of medicine is to preserve autonomy and that preservation of life is subservient to the primary goal" (Cassell 1977, 18). As we have seen, Cassell now believes it is the relief of suffering that constitutes the goal of medicine. Cassell wrote, in 1991, "There is some evidence that a single-minded concern with autonomy is beginning to pass from the bioethics scene" (Cassell 1991, 27).

11. This is a move that Engelhardt makes too. His rationale, we will see, is different than Royce's. For Engelhardt, autonomy is the central value of a secular humanist moral community because autonomous consent is the only possible basis for such a community.

12. "Intention" should be distinguished from "intentionality." The latter is a much broader term, originally used by Brentano to designate the quality (reference to an object) differentiating the psychological from the physical. It applies not only to intentions, but to beliefs, desires, and other psychological attitudes.

13. Royce, as a fallibilist, would hold: (1) that it is possible that his conception of loyalty, with the attendant notions of autonomy and well being, is flawed and (2) that even a clinician who is well trained in the philosophy of loyalty is susceptible to error in his assessment of the loyalty of his patients.

14. Engelhardt cannot turn this around by charging that the burden of proof is on Royce. Engelhardt specifically claims that every argument for content-full moral communities is based on arbitrary premises. Royce holds that his argument for establishing the great community is soundly based on an analysis of the nature of human moral agency, a basis that is hardly arbitrary. If Royce is correct, he negates Engelhardt's whole project.

15. My argument here is in no way designed to support the thesis of psychic determinism. Such a position would be disastrous to the interests of any moral community. Royce, along with Peirce, argues that initiative (spontaneity) is a differentiable characteristic of thought (OP, 42–46).

16. This is not to say that Royce would recommend violence or civil disobedience. These avenues would be reserved for the most extreme cases. However, he does expect the loyalist to speak up for his cause.

17. Engelhardt does, of course, introduce content into his skeletal system, recognizing that medicine is a practice, with built-in values. But he is always striving to give a minimalist account of these values.

Chapter 7

1. Of course, the argument has been put forth by thinkers such as Adam Smith and Milton Friedman that the social utility of free enterprise derives precisely from the fact that businesses pursue profit above all else. This "invisible hand" argument has been adequately dispatched on many occasions and does not warrant consideration in this book, except to note that it is especially ineffective against thinkers such as Royce, who do not measure social welfare in terms of economic productivity, consumption, or pleasure.

2. Dr. Williams related this story during a meeting at the 1993 ACEP Scientific Assembly. His comments are available on tape, through ACEP. The tape is entitled "Key Public Policy Issues for Emergency Medicine: The Next Five Years."

3. Perhaps a new generation of health care executives interested in streamlining medical services will provide an even greater impetus to rigid standardization. My impression, however, is that the employment of evidence-based medical care standards is more feasible under the direction of business persons than under the direction of politicians. If not, government oversight might actually be preferable to tight control of medical practice by profit-oriented businesses. Presumably, government leaders are more devoted than entrepreneurs to serving public interests.

4. Many of my observations here reflect those of Kadar ("The Sex Bias Myth in Medicine" in the August 1994 issue of *Atlantic Monthly*). I do not, of course, have room here for the extensive treatment of these issues that Kadar provides in his article.

5. We are finding that managed care, even apart from government oversight, may breed bureaucratic waste and may impede patient liberties. Also, profiteering may corrupt current pharmaceutical research to a greater degree than we would expect if this research were controlled by the government. Should these trends continue, my arguments against government intrusion will be undermined significantly. In any event, I believe that a strong case against for-profit health care corporations can already be made. The managers of investor-owned corporations have a fiduciary responsibility to shareholders. In health care, this obligation to primarily profit-oriented investors is apt to corrupt the service to the greater medical community.

6. I am increasingly skeptical about the role of for-profit health care corporations, though it is certainly true that "nonprofit" corporations are frequently interested in maximizing certain types of profit (for instance, those that pertain to the earnings of managers and physicians, or to the prospect of expanding facilities or services).

7. The notion of Medical Savings Accounts (MSAs) could be fruitful, not only as a method of stimulating frugality among patients who directly or indirectly purchase health insurance but also as an aspect of welfare reform.

8. There are several major problems with the notion of making antibiotics available without prescription. One is the emergence of antibiotic resistance. A second is the increased incidence of harmful effects of antibiotics, including serious disorders such as Stevens-Johnson syndrome, toxic epidermal necrolysis and pseudomembranous colitis. Finally, the inappropriate use of antibiotics can lead to a dangerous delay in diagnosis and a muddled clinical presentation in case of illnesses like bacterial meningitis. These objections do not pertain to the proposal that persons be allowed to purchase a rapid strep test and use positive results as a voucher to qualify them for the purchase of a 10-day supply of penicillin or erythromycin. Alternatively, the tests could be administered in the pharmacy.

9. DRGs, or diagnostic-related groups, is a program by which medical services are remunerated by diagnosis. A fixed sum of money is predetermined for every diagnosis. In such a system, the physician and hospital are able to make a profit only if they are able to treat the patient for less money than they will receive for the diagnosis. If not, they stand to lose money. As an intern, I recall being asked by a clerk to change a diagnosis from "acute renal failure" to "acute tubular necrosis" (or perhaps vice versa) for the sake of DRG reimbursement.

10. And also because she is a prospective member of the great community.

11. It is quite possible that I have learned more about loyalty by being married than I have by reading Royce.

12. For instance, if he made a habit out of withholding relatively expensive thera-

pies that would be of great enough benefit that their expense did not offset their overall benefit to society.

13. In their most recent book, *The Virtues in Medical Practice*, Pellegrino and Thomasma write, "We will concentrate on the imperative most central to being a profession and indispensable for medical morality—*effacement of self-interest*" (1993, 42).

14. Of course, the opinion here stated does not obligate me to a position on either side of the debate about assisted suicide. This issue does not hinge on the notion of medical futility. Instead, it hinges on questions about the meaning of certain forms of human existence and about what should come under the purview of medical "care." Royce would be helpful here, I believe. But I will not tackle this issue now.

15. According to this latter definition, there is nothing that keeps the most diverse varieties of moral theorist (or anti-theorist) from engaging in narrative ethics.

16. To their credit, these authors discuss the goals of medicine (Jonsen, Siegler, and Winslade 1992, 17), but they do not undergird these goals with a theory such as Royce's.

Chapter 8

1. Recall the letter to Elizabeth Randolph.

2. May's central image, that of the covenantor, has a biblical heritage.

3. Royce's notion of loyalty is itself largely metaphoric. The metaphoric character of moral theories has been investigated competently and provocatively by Mark Johnson and George Lakoff (Johnson and Lakoff 1980; Johnson 1993). Johnson argues in *Moral Imagination* (1993, 63–77) that all moral theories are grounded in metaphor, treating Kant's abstract and ostensibly nonmetaphoric ethical theory as a case in point. He seems to go astray, however, when he claims that our moral notion of "purpose" is mapped from the notion of a "destination," which occupies a more primary, physical "source" domain. Royce would counter that the notion of a destination would be incoherent apart from some kind of framework of purposes. In like fashion, many of Johnson's metaphors would be reversed by Royce, who would claim that certain moral notions are more primary than the physical correlates.

4. See Arthur Kleinman, *The Illness Narratives* for a provacative collection of medical stories.

5. Cabot's discussion of the use of placebos is also worth reading (1938, 148–150).

6. On the other hand, I would also refrain from claiming that the military metaphor is appropriate only for men, or for particularly masculine practitioners. There is, no doubt, something inherently masculine about combat. But, as the reader should apprehend through my employment of several Japanese concepts—such as *zuki no kokoro*, or "mind like the moon"—the male sexual metaphor (centering on penetration) is not the sole basis for military terminology. In the East, there is a profound appreciation for the manner in which great warriors instantiate polar elements of aggressiveness and passivity, bending and yielding, initiation and response, chaos and structure, frenzy and calm.

7. In Western thought, the concept of "inner harmony" applied to one in battle seems misplaced. This is not the case in the East. One of the most venerable of Japanese martial arts is *Aikido*, characterized as "the way of grace and harmony."

8. *Fingerspitzengefuhl* is best translated as "subtle intuition." Literally, it means "fingertip sense."

9. The original Chinese term from which "*mushin*" is derived is "*wu hsin.*" It is discussed by Merton in *Mystics and Zen Masters* (1961, 17–18).

10. There is similarity between this approach and Rosenzweig's technique, which utilizes neurolinguistic programming (NLP). The goal of NLP, according to Rosenzweig (1993), is to help the patient to "reframe" illness in more positive terms. NLP, however, does not specify what should count as "positive." See Trotter 1995, 381.

Bibliography

ACEP. 1993. "Clinical Policy for the Initial Approach to Children Under the Age of 2 Years Presenting with Fever." *Annals of Emergency Medicine* 22: 628–637.

——. 1994. "Changing Health Care Environment Leads to Development of "Standards of Care"." *ACEP News* 13: 13.

Ackernecht, E. W. 1955. *Short History of Medicine.* New York: Ronald Press Company.

Annas, George J. 1993. *Standard of Care: The Law of American Bioethics.* New York: Oxford University Press.

Aristotle. 1941. *The Basic Works of Aristotle.* Edited by Richard McKeon. New York: Random House.

——. 1962. *Nichomachean Ethics.* Translated by Martin Ostwald. Indianapolis: Bobbs-Merrill.

Ashley, Benedict M., and Kevin D. O'Rourke. 1989. *Health Care Ethics: A Theological Analysis.* 3d edition. St. Louis: The Catholic Health Association of the United States.

Baraff, L. J., et al. 1993. "Practice Guideline for the Management of Infants and Children 0 to 36 Months of Age with Fever without Source." *Annals of Emergency Medicine* 22: 1198–1210.

Baraff, L. J.; P. L.; Oppenheim; G. Sotriopoulos. 1994. "Incorporating Patient Preference into Practical Guidelines: Management of Children with Fever without Source." Abstract for the 5th International Conference on Emergency Medicine, London, England, May 23–26. *Annals of Emergency Medicine* 23: 923.

Bartelds, A. I. M., et. al. 1993. "Acute Otitis Media in Adults: A Report from the International Primary Care Network." *Journal of the American Board of Family Practice* 6: 333–339.

Bateson, G.; D. Jackson.; J. Haley; J. Weakland. 1956. "Towards a Theory of Schizophrenia." *Behavioral Science* 1: 251–264.

Baumeister, Roy F. 1986. *Identity: Cultural Change and the Struggle for Self.* New York: Oxford University Press.

Baumeister, Roy F.; Jeremy P. Shapiro; Diane M. Tice. 1985. "Two Kinds of Identity Crisis." *Journal of Personality* 53: 407–424.

Beauchamp, Tom L.; James F. Childress. 1979. *Principles of Biomedical Ethics.* New York: Oxford University Press.

Becker, H. S.; B. Geer, 1958. "The Fate of Idealism in Medical School." *Ameican Sociological Review* 23: 50–56.

Bradford, Ernle. 1972. *The Knights of the Order.* New York: Dorset Press.

Brody, Baruch A. 1988. *Life and Death Decision Making*. Oxford: Oxford University Press.

Brody, Howard. 1992. "The Importance of Primary Care for Theoretical Medicine: A Commentary." *Theoretical Medicine* 13(3): 261–263.

———. 1994. "My Story is Broken; Can You Help Me Fix It?" *Literature and Medicine* 13(1): 79–92.

Bukata, W. Richard. 1994. "The Enigma of Otitis Media." *Emergency Medicine and Acute Care Essays*.

Burns, Chester R. 1977. "Richard Clark Cabot (1868–1939) and Reformation in American Medical Ethics." *Bulletin of the History of Medicine* 51: 353–368.

Burton, Thomas W. 1994. "Caremark Faces Heat for Paying Doctors Who Sent It Patients." *Wall Street Journal*, November 11, A1.

Cabot, Richard Clark. 1914. *What Men Live By*. Boston: Houghton Mifflin.

———. 1916. "Josiah Royce as a Teacher." *Philosophical Review* 25: 466–472.

———. 1931. "Medical Ethics in the Hospital." *Nosokomeion* 2: 151–159.

———. 1932. "The Hospital as a Social Institution." *Nosokomeion* 3: 218–222.

———. 1933. *The Meaning of Right and Wrong*. New York: Macmillan.

———. 1936. *The Art of Ministering to the Sick*. New York: Macmillan.

———. 1938. *Honesty*. New York: Macmillan.

Camenisch, Paul F. 1992. "Business Ethics: On Getting to the Heart of the Matter." In *Moral Issues in Business*. Edited by William H. Shaw and Vincent Barry, 253–259. Belmont, Calif.: Wadsworth.

Camus, Albert. 1948. *The Plague*. Translated by Stuart Gilbert. New York: Modern Library.

———. 1955. *The Myth of Sisyphus*. Translated by Justin O'Brien. New York: Vintage.

Cassell, Eric J. 1977. "The Function of Medicine." *Hastings Center Report*, December, 16–19.

———. 1991. *The Nature of Suffering*. New York: Oxford University Press.

Christie, R.; R. K. Merton, 1958. "Procedures for the Sociological Study of the Value Climate in Medical Schools." *Journal of Medical Education* 33: 125–153.

Clendenning, John. 1985. *The Life and Thought of Josiah Royce*. Madison: University of Wisconsin Press.

Clouser, K. Danner; Bernard. Gert, 1990. "A Critique of Principlism." *Journal of Medicine and Philosophy* 15: 219–236.

Colwill, Jack M. 1992. "Where Have All the Primary Care Applicants Gone?" *New England Journal of Medicine* 326: 387–393.

Cotton, James Harry. 1954. *Royce on the Human Self*. Cambridge: Harvard University Press.

Cronin, A. J. [1937] 1965. *The Citadel*. Boston: Little, Brown and Company.

Dante. 1981. *Inferno*. Translated with an Introduction by Allen Mandelbaum. New York: Bantam.

Davis, Michael. "Explaining Wrongdoing." 1992. In *Moral Issues in Business*. Edited by William H. Shaw and Vincent Barry, 45–54. Belmont, Calif.: Wadsworth.

Dewey, John. 1934. *A Common Faith*. New Haven: Yale University Press.

———. 1977. *John Dewey: The Essential Writings*. Edited by David Sidorsky. New York: Harper & Row, 1977.

———. 1988. *Human Nature and Conduct*. Carbondale and Edwardsville: Southern Illinois University Press.

Dietrich, A. M., et al. 1993. "Pediatric Head Injuries: Can Clinical Factors Reliably Predict an Abnormality on Computed Tomography?" *Annals of Emergency Medicine* 22: 1535–1540.

Dolan, J. G., et al. 1993. "Diagnostic Strategies in the Management of Acute Upper Gastrointestinal Bleeding: Patient and Physician Preferences." *Journal of General Internal Medicine* 8: 525–529.

Dubovsky, Steven L. 1986. "Coping with Entitlement in Medical Education." *New England Journal of Medicine* 315: 1672–1674.

Duus, Benn R., et al. 1994. "The Role of Neuroimaging in the Initial Management of Patients with Minor Head Injury." *Annals of Emergency Medicine* 23: 1279–1283.

Dworkin, Gerald. 1976. "Autonomy and Behavior Control." *Hastings Center Report*, February, 23–28.

Engelhardt, H. Tristram, Jr. 1986. *The Foundations of Bioethics*. Oxford: Oxford University Press.

Eron, L. D. 1958. "The Effect of Medical Education on Attitudes: A Followup Study." *Journal of Medical Education* 33: 25–33.

Falk, Allan, and Alan Cohn. 1982. "Refining the Standard of Care: A Medicolegal Imperative." *Medical Trial Technique Quarterly* 29: 214–228.

Fischer, Louis. 1954. *Gandhi: His Life and Message for the World*. New York: Mentor.

Fletcher, George P. 1933. *Loyalty*. Oxford: Oxford University Press.

Fox, R. C. 1957. "Training for Uncertainty." In *The Student Physician*. Edited by R. K. Merton, G. Reader, and P. L. Kendall, 207–241. Cambridge, Mass.: Harvard University Press.

Fraser, David. 1993. *Knight's Cross*. New York: HarperCollins.

Friedman, Milton. 1962. *Capitalism and Freedom*. Chicago: University of Chicago Press.

Fuss, Peter. 1965. *The Moral Philosophy of Josiah Royce*. Cambridge: Harvard University Press.

Gandhi, Mohandas K. 1983. *Autobiography: The Story of My Experiments with Truth*. Translated by Mahadev Desai. New York: Dover.

Gantz, Jeffrey, trans. 1981. *Early Irish Myths and Sagas*. New York: Penguin.

Garrison, Fielding H. [1929] 1960. *An Introduction to the History of Medicine*. 4th edition. Philadelphia: W. B. Saunders.

Gaylin, Willard. 1978. "The Patient's Bill of Rights." In *Bioethics and Human Rights*. Edited by Elsie L. Bandman and Bertram Bandman, 265–267. Boston: Little, Brown and Company.

Gert, Bernard. [1966] 1988. *Morality: A New Justification of the Moral Rules*. Oxford: Oxford University Press.

Goldstein, E. 1979. "Psychological Adaptations of Soviet Immigrants." *American Journal of Psychoanalysis* 39: 257–263.

Greer, Thomas H. 1982. *A Brief History of the Western World*. 4th edition. New York: Harcourt Brace Jovanovich.

Gunther, John. 1949. *Death Be Not Proud*. New York: HarperPerennial.

Habermas, Jürgen. 1973. *Legitimation Crisis*. Translated by Thomas McCarthy. Boston: Beacon.

Harad, F. T., and M. D. Kerstein. 1992. "Inadequacy of Bedside Clinical Indicators in Identifying Significant Intracranial Injury in Trauma Patients." *Journal of Trauma* 32: 359–363.

Hocking, William Ernest. 1912. *The Meaning of God in Human Experience*. New Haven: Yale University Press.

———. 1937. *The Lasting Elements of Individualism*. New Haven: Yale University Press.

Hodges, Michael P. 1981. "Professional Ethics: Two Models for Understanding." Paper presented at the 11th annual conference of the American Society of Engineering Education, in Rapid City, South Dakota.

Holloway, Marguerite. 1994. "Trends in Women's Health: A Global View." *Scientific American* 271 (August): 76–83.

Howell, John M., et al. 1994. "Disposition, Discharge, and Follow-up." *Foresight* 30 (April): 1–8.

Humbach, Karl-Theo. 1962. *Das Verhältnis von Einzelperson und Gemeinschaft nach Josiah Royce*. Heidelberg: Carl Winter, Universitätsverlag. Translations are mine.

Iserson, Kenneth V.; Arthur B. Sanders; Deborah R. Mathieu; Allen E. Buchanan, eds. 1986. *Ethics in Emergency Medicine*. Baltimore: Williams & Wilkins.

James, William. [1967] 1977. *The Writings of William James*. Edited by John J. McDermott. Chicago: University of Chicago Press.

Jarvis, Edward A. 1975. *The Conception of God in the Later Royce*. The Hague: Martinus Nijhoff.

Johnson, Mark, and George Lackoff. 1980. *Metaphors We Live By*. Chicago: University of Chicago Press.

Johnson, Mark. *Moral Imagination*. 1993. Chicago: University of Chicago Press.

Jonsen, Albert R., and Stephen Toulmin. 1988. *The Abuse of Casuistry*. Berkeley: University of California Press.

Jonsen, Albert R. 1990. *The New Medicine and the Old Ethics*. Cambridge: Harvard University Press.

Jonsen, Albert R; Mark Siegler; William J. Winslade. 1992. *Clinical Ethics*. 3d edition New York: McGraw-Hill.

Kadar, Andrew G. 1994. "The Sex-Bias Myth in Medicine." *Atlantic Monthly* 274 (August): 66–70.

Kegley, Jacquelyn. 1993. "Today's Moral Imperative: Building Self and Community." Presented at Spring meeting of the Society for the Advancement of American Philosophy. Nashville, Tennessee.

———. 1997. *Genuine Individuals and Genuine Communities: A Roycean Public Philosophy*. Nashville: Vanderbilt University Press.

Kierkegaard, Søren. 1941. *Fear and Trembling; The Sickness Unto Death*. Translated and edited by Walter Lowrie. Princeton, N J.: Princeton University Press.

———. 1987. *Either/Or*. Translated and edited by Howard V. Hong and Edna H. Hong. Princeton, N.J.: Princeton University Press.

King, Ralph T., Jr. 1996. "How a Drug Firm Paid for University Study, Then Undermined It." *Wall Street Journal*, April 25, A1.

Kleinman, Arthur. 1988. *The Illness Narratives*. New York: Basic.

Kuklick, Bruce. 1972. *Josiah Royce: An Intellectual Biography*. Indianapolis: Bobbs-Merrill.

Lachs, John. 1981. *Intermediate Man*. Indianapolis: Hackett.

———. 1995. *The Relevance of Philosophy to Life*. Nashville: Vanderbilt University Press.

Larson, James. 1996. "Don't Trust Salary Surveys." *Unique Opportunities* 6(3): 54–56.

Leonard, George. 1991. *Mastery*. New York: Dutton.

Levi, D. L.; H. Stierlin; R. J. Savard. 1972. "Fathers and Sons: The Interlocking Crises of Integrity and Identity." *Psychiatry* 35: 48–56.

Locke, John. [1690] 1980. *Second Treatise of Government*. Edited by C. B. Macpherson. Indianapolis: Hackett.

MacIntyre, Alasdair. 1981. *After Virtue*. Notre Dame, Ind.: University of Notre Dame Press.

———. 1988. *Whose Justice? Which Rationality?* Notre Dame, Ind.: University of Notre Dame Press.

———. 1990. *Three Rival Versions of Moral Enquiry*. Notre Dame, Ind.: University of Notre Dame Press.

Mahowald, Mary B. 1972. *An Idealistic Pragmatist: The Development of the Pragmatic Element in the Philosophy of Josiah Royce*. The Hague: Martinus Nijhoff.

Marcel, Gabriel. [1956] 1975. Reprint. *Royce's Metaphysics*. Translated by Gordon Ringer and Virginia Ringer. Westport, Connecticut: Greenwood Press. .

Marx, Karl. 1963. *Karl Marx: Early Writings*. Translated by T. B. Bottomore. New York: McGraw-Hill.

May, William F. 1983. *The Physician's Covenant*. Phildelphia: Westminster.

Mead, George Herbert. 1982. *Selected Writings of George Herbert Mead*. Edited by Andrew Reck. Chicago: University of Chicago Press.

Merton, Thomas. 1961. *Mystics and Zen Masters*. New York: Noonday Press.

Mill, John Stuart. [1861] 1957. *Utilitarianism*. Edited by Oskar Piest. Indianapolis: Bobbs-Merrill.

Mohanty, S. K.; W. Thompson; S. Rakower. 1991. "Are CT Scans For Head Injury Patients Always Necessary?" *Journal of Trauma* 31: 801–804.

Morreim, E. Haavi. 1991. *Balancing Act: The New Medical Ethics of Medicine's New Economics*. Boston: Kluwer Academic Publishers.

Mostwin, D. 1976. "Uprootment and Anxiety." *International Journal of Mental Health* 5: 103–116.

Mowrer, O. Hobart. 1961. *The Crisis in Psychiatry and Religion*. New York: D. Van Nostrand.

Miyamoto, Musashi. 1993. *The Book of Five Rings*. Translated by Thomas Cleary. Boston: Shambhala.

Nelson, Hilda Lindemann. 1992. "Against Caring." *The Journal of Clinical Ethics* 3(1): 8–15.

———. 1995. "What's Narrative Ethics?" *Center View* 4(2): 1–2.

Nietzsche, Friedrich. 1966. *Beyond Good and Evil*. Translated by Walter Kaufmann. New York: Vintage.

———. 1966. *Thus Spoke Zarathustra*. Translated by Walter Kaufmann. New York: Penguin.

Noddings, Nel. 1984. *Caring: A Feminine Approach to Ethics and Moral Education*. Berkeley: University of California Press.

———. 1992. "In Defense of Caring." *The Journal of Clinical Ethics* 3(1): 15–18.

Nozick, Robert. 1974. *Anarchy, State, and Utopia*. New York: Basic Books.

Nuland, Sherwin B. 1988. *Doctors: The Biography*. New York: Vintage.

Oppenheim, Frank M. 1987. *Royce's Mature Philosophy of Religion*. Notre Dame, Ind.: Notre Dame University Press.

———. 1989. "A Roycean Response to Individualism." In *Beyond Individualism: Toward a Retrieval of Moral Discourse in America*. Edited by Donald L. Gelpi, 87–119. Notre Dame, Ind.: University of Notre Dame Press.

———. 1993. *Royce's Mature Ethics*. Notre Dame, Ind.: Notre Dame University Press, 1993.

———. 1994. "Four Practical Challenges of the Mature Royce to Californians and Others." *Transactions of the Charles S. Peirce Society* 30: 803–824.

Osler, William. 1932. *Aequanimitas*. 3d edition. Philadelphia: Blakiston.

Parker, Sheryl L.; Tony Tong, Sherry Bolden, Phyllis A. Wingo. "Cancer Statistics, 1996." *CA—A Cancer Journal for Clinicians* 46: 5–27.

Peirce, Charles Sanders. 1955. *Philosophical Writings of Peirce*. New York: Dover.

Pellegrino, Edmund D., and David C. Thomasma. 1988. *For the Patient's Good*. Oxford: Oxford University Press.

———. 1993. *The Virtues in Medical Practice*. New York: Oxford University Press.

Percival, Thomas. 1985. *Medical Ethics*. Birmingham, Ala.: Classics of Medicine Library.

Philibert, Owen. 1994. Letter to the Editor. *Sports Illustrated*, May 30. 8.

Plato. 1961. *The Collected Dialogues of Plato*. Edited by Edith Hamilton and Huntington Cairns. Princeton, N.J.: Princeton University Press.

Pollock, Ellen Joan. 1995. "Managed Care's Focus on Psychiatric Drugs Alarms Many Doctors." *Wall Street Journal*, December 1, A1.

Porter, Jean. 1993. "Openness and Constraint: Moral Reflection as Tradition-Guided Inquiry in Alasdair MacIntyre's Recent Works." *The Journal of Religion* 73: 514–536.

Reinus, W. R.; F. J. Wippold; K. E. Erickson. 1993. "Practical Selection Criteria for Noncontrast Cranial Computed Tomography in Patients with Head Trauma." *Annals of Emergency Medicine* 22: 1148–1155.

Rezler, Agnes G. 1974. "Attitude Changes During Medical School: A Review of the Literature." *Journal of Medical Education* 49: 1023–1030.

Rimel, R. W., and J. A. Jane. 1985. "Minor Head Injury: Management and Outcome." In *Neurosurgery*. Edited by R. H. Wilkins and S. S. Rengachary, 1608–1611. New York: McGraw-Hill.

Robinson, Daniel S. 1968. *Royce and Hocking: American Idealists*. Boston: Christopher.

Roeske, N. A., and K. Lake. 1977. "Role Models for Women Medical Students." *Journal of Medical Education* 52: 459–466.

Roosevelt, Theodore. 1903. *The Strenuous Life: Essays and Addresses*. New York: Century.

Rosenzweig, Steven. 1993. "Emergency Rapport." *Journal of Emergency Medicine* 11: 775–778.

Royce, Josiah. ca. 1883–1884. "Lectures on the History of Ethics." Harvard University Archives, Royce Papers, folio 89.

———. 1885. *The Religious Aspect of Philosophy*. Boston: Houghton Mifflin.

———. 1897. *The Conception of God*. New York: Macmillan.

———. 1900. *The Conception of Immortality*. Boston: Houghton Mifflin.

———. [1901] 1976. *The World and the Individual*. Gloucester, Mass.: Peter Smith. 2 vols.

———. 1903. *Outlines of Psychology*. New York: Macmillan.

———. 1904. *Herbert Spencer: An Estimate and a Review*. New York: Fox, Duffield.

———. 1906. *Studies in Good and Evil*. New York: D. Appleton and Company.

———. [1908] 1995. Reprint. *The Philosophy of Loyalty*. Introduction by John J. McDermott. Nashville: Vanderbilt University Press.

———. 1908. *Race Questions and Other American Problems*. New York: Macmillan.

———. 1908. Pittsburgh lectures on the doctrine of loyalty. Harvard University Archives, Royce Papers, folio 82.

———. 1911. *William James and Other Essays on the Philosophy of Life*. New York: Macmillan.

———. 1912. *The Sources of Religious Insight*. New York: Charles Scribners's Sons.

———. 1914. *War and Insurance*. New York: Macmillan.

———. 1915–1916. Extension Course on Ethics. Harvard University Archives, Royce Papers, folios 94 and 95.

———. 1916. *The Hope of the Great Community*. New York: Macmillan.

———. [1918] 1968. Reprint. *The Problem of Christianity*. Introduction by John E. Smith. Chicago: University of Chicago Press.

———. 1951. *Royce's Logical Essays*. Edited by Daniel S. Robinson. Dubuque: William C. Brown.

———. 1967. "Royce's Urbana Lectures: Lecture II." Edited by Peter Fuss. *Journal of the History of Philosophy* V(3): 269–286.

———. 1970. *The Letters of Josiah Royce*. Edited by John Clendenning. Chicago: Chicago University Press.

Safire, William. 1992. *Lend Me Your Ears*. New York: W.W. Norton.

Saloman, Bonnie. 1994. "Morals and Mortals in the Emergency Department." *Annals of Emergency Medicine* 23: 124–125.

Schoeneweis, Barbara J., and James E. George. 1992. "A Secret Risk Management Weapon: Customer Service in the Emergency Department." *Emergency Physician Legal Bulletin* 3: 1–8.

Schopenhauer, Arthur. [1883] 1969. Reprint. *The World as Will and Representation*. 2 vols. Translated by E. F. J. Payne. New York: Dover, 1969.

Schweitzer, Albert. 1965. *A Treasury of Albert Schweitzer*. Edited by Thomas Kiernan. New York: Gramercy.

Shackford, Steven R., et al. 1992. "The Clinical Utility of Computed Tomographic Scanning and Neurological Examination in the Management of Patients with Minor Head Injuries." *Journal of Trauma* 33: 385–394.

Shaw, William H., and Vincent Barry. 1992. *Moral Issues in Business*. 5th Edition. Belmont, Calif.: Wadsworth.

Shem, Samuel. 1978. *The House of God*. New York: Dell.

Sigerist, Henry E. 1951. *A History of Medicine*. New York: Oxford University Press.

Smith, John E. [1950] 1969. *Royce's Social Infinite*. Hamden, Conn.: Archon Books.

Smith, Earl E. 1993. "Variations in Clinical Guidelines." *Annals of Emergency Medicine* 22: 1196–1197.

Stein, S. C., and S. E. Ross. 1993. "Minor Head Injury: A Proposed Strategy for Emergency Management." *Annals of Emergency Medicine* 22: 1193–1196.

Stern, Daniel N. 1985. *The Interpersonal World of the Infant*. New York: Basic.

Swift, E. M. 1994. "Give Young Athletes a Fair Shake." *Sports Illustrated*, May 2, 76.

Trotter, Griffin. 1994. "Royce, Community and Ethnicity." *Transactions of the Charles S. Peirce Society* 30: 231–269.

————. 1995. "The Loyal Physician: An Essay Applying the Ethics of Josiah Royce to the Practice of Medicine." Ph.D. dissertation. Vanderbilt University.

Turnbull, Stephen. 1989. *Samurai Warlords: The Book of Daimy.* London: Blandford.

Veatch, Robert M. 1981. *A Theory of Medical Ethics.* New York: Basic.

West, Cornel. 1993. *Keeping Faith.* New York: Routledge.

Young, Debra D. 1988–1989. "The Idaho Standard of Care in Medical Malpractice Cases." *Idaho Law Review* 25: 415–25.

Zaner, Richard M. 1988. *Ethics and the Clinical Encounter.* Englewood Cliffs, N.J.: Prentice Hall.

————. 1993. "Voices and Time: The Venture of Clinical Ethics." *Journal of Medicine and Philosophy* 18: 9–31.

Index

Griffin Trotter holds an M.D. degree from St. Louis University and a Ph.D. from Vanderbilt University in American philosophy. He has worked for ten years as an emergency physician, in a variety of settings, and presently is assistant professor of ethics at the Center for Health Care Ethics, St. Louis University Health Sciences Center.

THE LOYAL PHYSICIAN

was composed electronically
using Adobe Garamond types, with displays in
Adobe Garamond Expert, Adobe Garamond Titling,
and Zapf Dingbats. The book was printed on Natural Smooth
acid-free, recycled paper and was Smyth sewn and cased in Roxite B-grade
cloth over 88-point binder's boards, head bands, and matching end leaves,
with dust jackets printed in two colors by Braun-Brumfield, Inc.
Both book and jacket design are the work of Gary Gore.
Published by Vanderbilt University Press
Nashville, Tennessee 37235